FOOTBALL TRAINING

FOR THE ATHLETE, BY THE ATHLETE

TRIUMPH
B O O K S

This book is available in quantity at special discounts for your group or organization. For further information, contact:
Triumph Books
542 South Dearborn Street
Suite 750
Chicago, Illinois 60605
(312) 939–3330
Fax (312) 663–3557
www.triumphbooks.com

Printed in India
ISBN: 978-1-60078-280-0

Design, page production, and editing: Red Line Editorial

Contributing Writers:
Chad Zimmerman
Josh Staph
Chip Smith
Scott Mackar
Zac Clark
Matt Siracusa
Kyle Woody

Photos courtesy STACK Media unless otherwise indicated.

ABOUT STACK

STACK is the nation's leading producer and distributor of sports performance, training, and lifestyle content for high school and college athletes and the high school sports community. Founded by Nick Palazzo and Chad Zimmerman, two former collegiate football athletes, STACK has the singular goal of improving the lives of athletes by providing safe and effective advice on how to properly boost performance without the use of steroids or other illegal performance-enhancing drugs.

The name STACK stands for the complete "stack" of information an athlete needs to be more successful in all aspects of life. Key components are STACK's information, instruction, and advice on training and nutrition that help athletes improve their physical being and performance. But STACK also addresses important life skills and teaches lessons in areas such as team building, goal setting, mental preparation, and overcoming adversity. Finally, a very important part of STACK's content mix is material related to college selection and the recruiting process, including tips and advice on character building, presenting oneself properly to coaches, and focusing on strong academics.

STACK's content does not come from individuals who claim to be "experts," but have little experience working with elite athletes. On the contrary, the information and advice provided by STACK comes directly from today's best athletes and the experts who work with them on a regular basis. Athletes such as Peyton Manning, LeBron James, Johan Santana, LaDainian Tomlinson, Allen Iverson, and Tim Duncan have willingly made their training, nutrition, or personal experiences available to STACK's audience. Why? Because they want to support STACK's mission of helping athletes safely improve their performance. By using star professional athletes as role models, STACK produces content that's real, raw, and authentic and makes a powerful and lasting impression on its readers and viewers.

CONTENTS

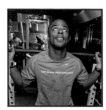

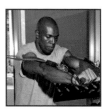

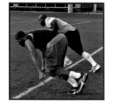

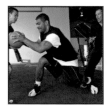

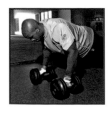

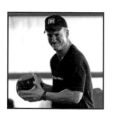
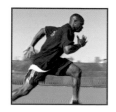
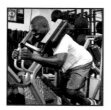
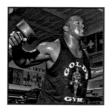
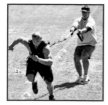

INTRODUCTION

How is this Book Different?

This book is a compilation of the best football workouts published in *STACK* Magazine since the company was launched 2005. Over the past four and a half years, *STACK* content directors have observed hundreds of workouts by some of the best professional and collegiate players and strength coaches in the business. In the following pages, you'll gain exclusive insights into how successful pros such as Adrian Peterson, Peyton Manning, LaDainian Tomlinson, and Brian Urlacher prepare their bodies to perform at peak levels during the long and demanding NFL season. Unlike those in some other publications, these workouts are real. They are the exact regimens used by each featured NFL star every day, week, month, and year. The impeccable, polished product you see on the field every Sunday is crafted—with little or no fanfare—in the gym, on the practice field, and on the track. If you want to know how these men were shaped into formidable athletes, read on.

What is STACK?

STACK is the nation's leading producer and distributor of sports performance, training, and lifestyle content for active sports participants.

Recognizing the need and in response to the demand for state-of-the-art sports performance information, former collegiate football players Nick Palazzo and Chad Zimmerman launched STACK in February 2005. Their singular goal was to improve the lives of young athletes by providing safe and effective advice on how to boost performance without the use of steroids or other illegal performance-enhancing drugs. Since the company's founding, the STACK editorial team, which produces all of the company's original content, has been forging relationships with the best and brightest in the sports performance, sports nutrition, strength and conditioning, recruiting, sports psychology, and related fields, all of which are vital to developing a well-rounded athlete. Via recorded interviews and video shoots, more than 400 experts have contributed to STACK's content library, providing readers and website visitors with easy access to the cutting-edge and groundbreaking techniques that help already-elite athletes get even better. This access is what separates STACK from other media properties and what makes STACK's content real, raw, and authentic.

STACK's Objectives

The three pillars of STACK's mission to athletes are to provide:

- Information, instruction, and advice on training and nutrition that help athletes enhance physical well-being, improve on-field performance, and avoid injury
- Emphasis on important life skills that teach lessons in areas such as team building, goal setting, mental preparation, and overcoming adversity

- Advice on the college selection and recruiting process, including tips and suggestions on character building, presenting oneself properly to coaches, and focusing on strong academics.

STACK Platforms

STACK reaches its ever-expanding audience through STACK Media, *STACK* Magazine, STACK.com, STACK TV, and MySTACK.

STACK Media is one of the top sports properties on the Internet, with an average of four million unique visitors and 100 million page views per month, according to comScore. Recognizing that active young males are hard to reach online, STACK Media combines its unique and appealing editorial content with product and service offerings from a number of related partner sites to fully engage its audience through a distributed media network. From its origins as a magazine publisher, STACK Media has become the acknowledged leader in reaching active sports participants online.

STACK Magazine, requested by more than 9,000 high school athletic directors, has a circulation of 800,000 and a readership of nearly five million high school athletes. In keeping with the company's mission, the magazine is devoted to helping shape well-rounded athletes. Published six times throughout the school year, the magazine is loaded with expert advice from top professional athletes and their trainers. *STACK* Magazine teaches young athletes the proper way to train, eat, and develop their skills, while also educating them on how to be good teammates, respect their opponents, and handle adversity—lessons based on the experiences of pro and college athletes who have reached the pinnacle of success in their sports.

STACK.com, the digital home for all STACK content and web-based tools, provides content exclusively for youth sports participants. With coverage of more than 20 sports and content featuring lifestyle information as well as training, nutrition, and sports skills, the site offers something for everyone with an interest in sports performance.

STACK TV, an online platform with eight channels and several categories of unique, proprietary videos, constitutes the largest video library of sports performance content on the web. More than 4,000 [and counting] videos feature top professional and collegiate athletes, coaches, trainers, and sports nutritionists, all offering the benefits of their expertise to young athletes seeking to improve their performance.

MySTACK is a social network and recruiting site that allows athletes to create profiles with their personal information and athletic stats, upload highlight films and photos, and send their profiles to college coaches. Tens of thousands of athletes have signed up as MySTACK members, and many use the network to connect [and compete] with each other as well as to take control of the recruiting process, confirming the proposition that competition breeds success.

STACK EXPERTS

CHIP SMITH
Competitive Edge Sports
Founder
competitiveedgesports.com

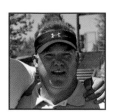

Considered one of the forefathers of
the sports training industry, Smith has
trained more than 300 NFL players
during his career. His impressive
football clientele, most of whom train at Smith's Competitive
Edge Sports facility [Duluth, Georgia], includes 39 Pro Bowl
players, 20 first-round draft picks, three Heisman Trophy
winners, and 25 NCAA All-Americans. A two-sport athlete
[football and baseball] at Liberty University, Smith still holds
rushing and scoring records. In the mid-1980s, he studied at
the famed Soviet Sports Institute upon invitation, and he has
headed the U.S. Olympic Power Lifting team.

DANNY ARNOLD
Plex
Owner
plex.cc

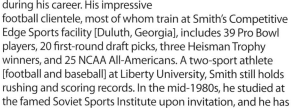

As the owner of Plex [Houston, Texas],
Arnold oversees all of the facility's
operations. His current clientele
includes NFL superstars Casey
Hampton, Julius Peppers, Shaun Rogers, and Olympic gold
medalist Steven Lopez. Arnold's staff includes performance
specialists, physical therapists, athletic trainers, doctors,
coaches, and former collegiate and professional athletes.
The Plex team replaces traditional sports training with
scientifically designed and technologically advanced
methods that train athletes on movements directly used
in their respective sports. Prior to opening Plex, Arnold
graduated with a bachelor of science from Texas Southern
University, where he played football and ran track. After
graduating, he served as a coach for the Tiger football and
track teams.

LUKE RICHESSON
Jacksonville Jaguars
Strength and conditioning coach
jaguars.com

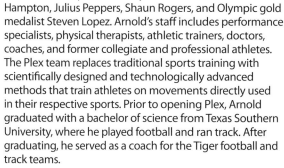

Richesson, a former performance
specialist at Athletes' Performance,
worked with future NFL stars Adrian
Peterson, Patrick Willis, and Alan
Branch before the 2007 NFL Combine. During his nine years
at AP, Richesson helped prepare more than 214 NFL draftees
for the rigorous combine. A former University of Kansas
football player, Richesson joined the Jacksonville Jaguars in
2009 as strength and conditioning coach.

ROBERT FITZPATRICK
Pittsburgh Steelers
Former assistant strength coach

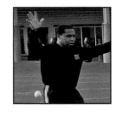

Fitzpatrick helped revitalize the
Pittsburgh Steelers' speed program
upon his hiring in 2004. A two-time
selection as one of *Men's Journal*'s Top
100 Trainers in America, Fitzpatrick
helped develop a speed program to enhance explosiveness
and first-step speed for all Steelers players, including
standouts Hines Ward and James Harrison.

TERRELL OWENS
Buffalo Bills
Wide receiver
buffalobills.com
Terrell Owens Enterprises
Founder
terrellowens.com

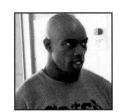

Better known as T.O., the Alabama
native honed his athletic skills at the University of Tennessee-
Chattanooga, where he thrived on the gridiron and
hardwood. Owens' dream of turning pro became a reality
when the San Francisco 49ers selected him 98th overall
during the third round of the 1996 NFL Draft. In 2004, he
signed as a free agent with the Philadelphia Eagles, and
two years later he joined the Dallas Cowboys. In 2008, he
published *T.O.'s Finding Fitness: Making the Mind, Body, and
Spirit Connection for Total Health*, which details workout
routines suitable for all levels and in- and off-season nutrition
guides. In March 2009, T.O. signed with the Buffalo Bills as a
free agent.

TODD DURKIN
Fitness Quest 10
Owner
fitnessquest10.com; todddurkin.com

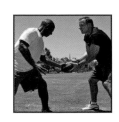

Durkin, owner and operator of
the Fitness Quest 10 facility [San
Diego, California], is a performance
enhancement specialist who works
with top professional, Olympic, and world-class athletes. His
clientele includes NFL players LaDainian Tomlinson, Drew
Brees, and Donnie Edwards, and major league pitcher Mark
Prior. Recognized as the Personal Trainer of the Year in 2004
by IDEA Health and Fitness Association and again in 2005 by
ACE, Durkin is a leading authority on human performance.
He gives lectures worldwide on a wide range of fitness
topics. Durkin's professional career as a quarterback was cut
short due to a severe back injury—an experience he uses to
produce training programs focused on injury prevention
and rehabilitation.

TOM SHAW

Tom Shaw Performance
Enhancement
Owner
coachtomshaw.com

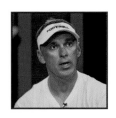

Shaw is one of the nation's top
speed and strength coaches. Best
known for improving NFL prospects'
draft stock, the SPARQ Master Trainer also specializes in
training the NFL's best in the off-season. He's worked with
more than 90 NFL first-round selections and seven Super
Bowl MVPs. Shaw served as the speed and conditioning
coach for the three-time Super Bowl champion New
England Patriots, and he held the same position prior
to that for six seasons with the New Orleans Saints. He
also spent eight seasons as an assistant track coach at
Florida State University, working primarily with sprinters
and jumpers. Shaw's past clients include Deion Sanders,
Peyton Manning, Tom Brady, and Reggie Bush.

TRAVELLE GAINES

Elite Athletics
Director, pro athlete development
eliteathletics.com

Gaines heads up day-to-day
operations and training at the
recently opened Elite Athletics in
Westlake Village, California. New
Orleans Saints tight end and 10-
year NFL veteran Billy Miller opened the state-of-the-art
facility in 2008 and brought in Gaines shortly thereafter.
Gaines has trained NFL and NBA players, including Marcus
Trufant [Seattle Seahawks 2008 Pro Bowl CB], Brandon
Roy [2006–2007 NBA Rookie of the Year], Lawyer Milloy
[14-year NFL vet], Jamal Crawford [New York Knicks
guard], and Willie Parker [Pittsburgh Steelers 2007, 2008
Pro Bowl RB]. Prior to his current position, Gaines worked
with the Jacksonville Jaguars' strength and conditioning
staff during training camp, and he was a strength and
conditioning coach at University of Louisiana–Monroe
and Louisiana State University, training first-round picks
Joseph Addai, JaMarcus Russell, Glenn Dorsey, LaRon
Landry, Dwayne Bowe, and Craig "Buster" Davis.

WILL BARTHOLOMEW

Explosion Sports, LLC [parent
company of D1 Sports Training and
Therapy]
President and CEO
d1sportstraining.com

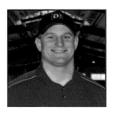

Bartholomew's passion and vision
for sports training led him to open
the first D1 Sports Training facility in a 1,000-square-foot
warehouse just outside Nashville in 2002. Since then, D1
has expanded across Tennessee to Memphis, Knoxville,
and Chattanooga. He's also opened facilities in Little Rock,
Arkansas, Huntsville, Alabama, and Greenville, South
Carolina. Bartholomew was a three-year starting fullback
at the University of Tennessee, serving as team captain
in 2001. As a Volunteer, he was twice named "Lifter of the
Year" and was president of the Fellowship of Christian
Athletes for three years. After graduation, he played for
the Denver Broncos until suffering a career-ending knee
injury. Through his time as a Volunteer, Bartholomew
formed a relationship with teammate Peyton Manning,
who now serves as co-owner of D1. Other D1 co-owners
include NFL quarterback Philip Rivers, NBA player Shane
Battier, and former undisputed middleweight champion
Jermain Taylor.

WILLIAM HICKS

Syracuse University
Assistant athletics director for
athletic performance
suathletics.com

At Syracuse University, Hicks is
responsible for the strength and
conditioning program for the
school's 21 intercollegiate athletic teams. He is also the
head strength and conditioning coach for the Orange
football program. Before heading to Syracuse in 2000,
Hicks held the following positions at North Carolina State
between 1986 and 2000: athletic improvement coach,
athletic improvement coordinator, director of athletic
improvement, and assistant athletic director for football
operations. During his 24-year career, he has contributed
to the development of NFL All-Pros Dwight Freeney and
Torry Holt, Super Bowl champions David Tyree and Anthony
Smith, and NFL first-round draft picks Will Allen, Haywood
Jeffries, and Dewayne Washington.

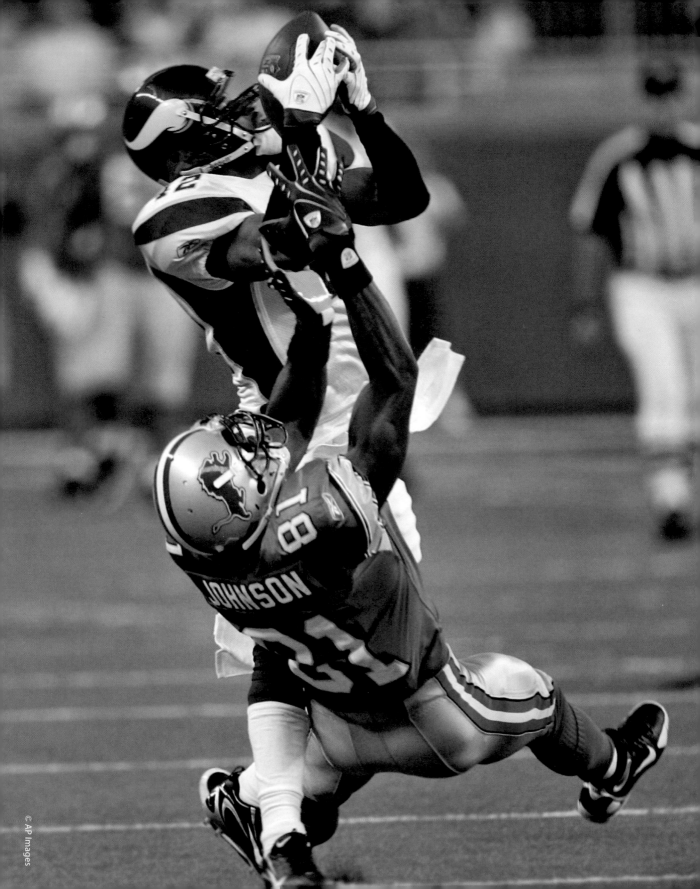

CHAPTER 1

DARREN SHARPER

EDITOR'S NOTE

In July 2007, we had the opportunity to spend a day at Disney's Wide World of Sports complex in Orlando, Florida, and to witness a workout directed by legendary sports performance coach Tom Shaw. Best known for his ability to help athletes improve their top-end and position-specific speed, Shaw has worked hands-on with an impressive list of pro athletes. Needless to say, we were thrilled at the chance to see how one of the best in the industry does his work.

On that hot and humid Florida afternoon, Shaw put his troops through an intense, efficient, and all-business workout, making it an easy decision for us to include it in our top 10 favorite football training sessions. More than 20 NFL athletes performed speed, agility, and reaction training, followed by intense weight room work. Although plenty of elite athletes were on location—including Pittsburgh Steelers Ike Taylor and James Farrior, fresh off their 2007 Super Bowl win—we focused on Pro Bowl safety Darren Sharper.

A longtime Shaw client, Sharper earned his first Pro Bowl bid in the campaign immediately following the first off-season during which he trained with the guru. From that point on, Sharper

DARREN SHARPER DEFENDS A PASS DURING A GAME AGAINST THE LIONS. SHARPER'S OFF-SEASON TRAINING REGIMEN HAS HELPED HIM STAY AT THE TOP OF THE GAME FOR MORE THAN A DECADE.

continued to train with Shaw to amp his game. Three more Pro Bowl appearances have followed in Sharper's storied career, during which he has cracked the top 20 in NFL history for career interceptions.

The following article, featured in the November/December 2007 issue of *STACK* Magazine, was based on the speed portion of Sharper's workout. However, we've also thrown in some never-before-seen photos of Sharper completing his weight room routine, which included squats, hang cleans, leg extensions, leg curls, single-leg squats, and various other lower-body exercises.

BIGGER, FASTER, STRONGER, SHARPER

Practice does not make perfect.

Perfect practice—working your hardest in game mode, in the off-season—makes perfect. It's a subtle distinction, but one that can mean the difference between all-star and benchwarmer.

Darren Sharper knows this.

Football training is pace-specific. That means the speed you train at during practice is the pace you'll use on the field during competition. So you'd better move as fast you can.

Most of the plays Sharper runs are at least 40 yards, times an average of 65 snaps in a game. "Just add all that up and see what you come up with," he urges. "It's a lot of running."

"And the time you don't run as fast as you can is the time you get beat. I can't afford that."

Sharper, who's built quite a reputation as a big-play guy, has certainly beaten the odds. With the average NFL career spanning just less than four years, the Pro Bowl player has played

11 NFL campaigns, and he just signed a new contract with the New Orleans Saints in 2009. He still looks and performs as good as ever, a testament to the value of his off-season training. He says, "Football is such a rigorous sport, you know? The training I've done off the field has provided my longevity."

It wasn't always like that for Sharper.

"As I continued to play, I realized that I suffered more injuries during the regular season if I didn't come into training camp in excellent shape," he says.

Many NFL players taper back their conditioning as they enter the season, but Sharper did the exact opposite. He upped his training intensity and sought out speed expert Tom Shaw, who has worked with 85 first-round NFL Draft choices and trained seven Super Bowl MVPs.

"Before my fourth season, I started to work with Coach Shaw on my speed and explosiveness," Sharper says. "That's when I really noticed a difference in my performance."

A great idea turned into a tradition for Sharper, who now heads to the Wide World of Sports in Orlando every off-season.

Enhancing both his finesse and raw strength, Sharper's training has enabled him to play both sides of the coin. Poised and ready to pounce, he can pull a pass out of mid-air, turning an interception into art. Back on defense, he can zone in on and smash into an unaware running back, causing a fumble.

"There are some situations when you just have to flat-out run a guy down," Sharper says.

Shaw's secret to helping Sharper's speed?

A simple bungee cord.

"Football is a game of angles," Shaw says. "The bungee cords and belts enable our guys to have 360-degree resistance. Every single step—whether it's the backpedal, turn or sprint—is trained with 20 percent resistance."

This allows the player to have more hip power and stride length, which, as Shaw points out, are essential to reaching top speed.

"The number-one thing is being explosive," Shaw says. "We work on pushing ourselves down the field. The longer your strides, the faster you'll run—period."

In football, a wasted movement or hesitation can spell the difference between winning and losing.

"The bungees pull you into a position really quickly," Shaw says. "[They force you] to get your feet right back underneath you, which is essential to cutting and breaking away."

Sharper fully understands the benefits of using the cords: "Once you take away the resistance of the cords, you feel a lot lighter and freer. Your body just takes off."

His only regret is that he didn't start using them sooner: "It's definitely something I would have done when I was younger. All through high school and up until my first few years of college, I just didn't take advantage of them."

Check out the bungee cord exercises Shaw uses to make Sharper a defensive threat.

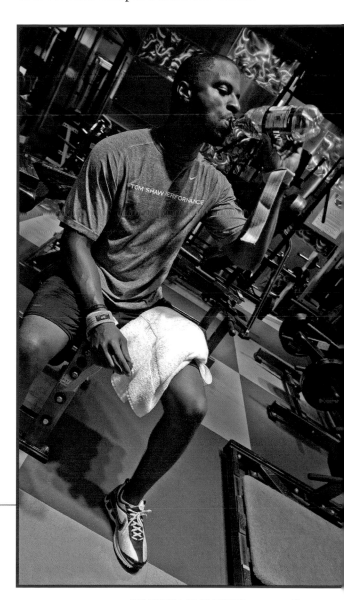

Bungee Cord Workout Tips

1. Safety First

"The bungee is one of the more dangerous exercises you'll do," Shaw says. "You don't want to feel like you're pulling a truck."

So, he recommends using only 20 percent resistance; that way you use the same form and technique you do on the field.

"You want to be in a position to be explosive," Sharper adds.

2. No Wasted Movements

According to Shaw, most athletes have a tendency to keep their bodies high when backpedaling, which is a wasted movement that slows them down.

"Once you rise out of your stance," Shaw says, "you have to get back into an acceleration position, which means dropping back down."

The bottom line? Stay low.

3. Maintain Proper Form

When backpedaling, Shaw recommends keeping your nose right over your toes and your head level, so you can turn and run smoothly at any angle.

"You have to make it perfect, because you don't want any separation from the receiver or the guy you're trying to cover," he explains.

Also, make sure to keep a slight forward lean and get your elbows pumping.

"The faster you move your elbows, the faster your feet go."

4. Get Adequate Rest Between Sets

"The harder you work the more rest you need," Shaw says. "I don't want my athletes feeling gassed before they run again."

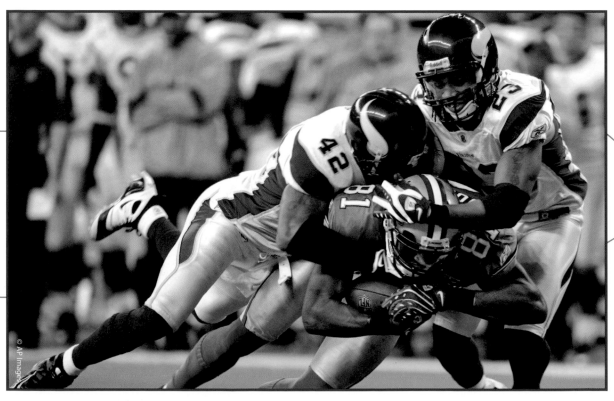

© AP Images

QUICK-FEET LADDER DRILLS

IN, BEHIND, OUT

- Step right foot into first box

- Swing left foot behind right foot while simultaneously lifting right foot

- Land with both feet outside of ladder to right so that right foot is in front of left

- Step left foot into next box; repeat sequence to opposite side

- Repeat continuously down length of ladder

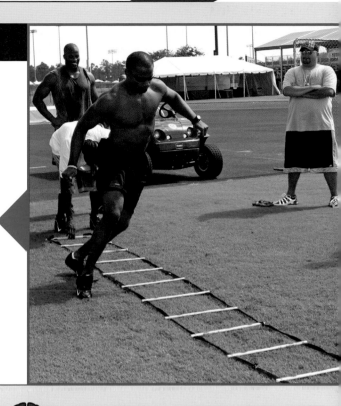

STRAIGHT-AHEAD SPRINT

- Sprint down length of ladder, placing one foot in each box with rapid high-knee motion

- Step right foot into first box

- Step left foot into first box

- Step right foot outside of ladder to right

- Step left foot outside of ladder to left

- Repeat sequence

- Continue down length of ladder thinking: "in, in, out, out"

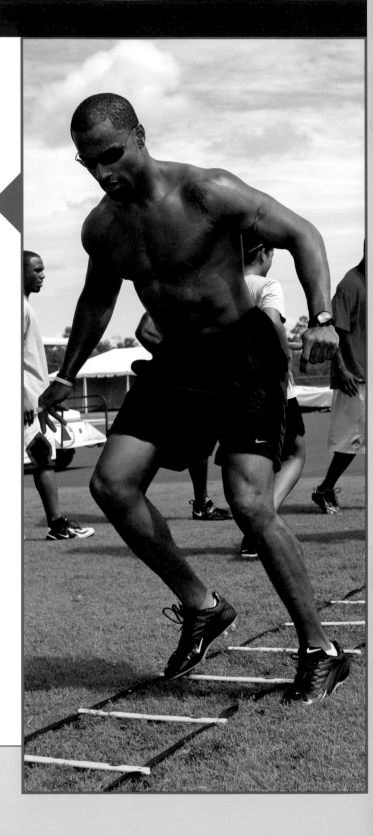

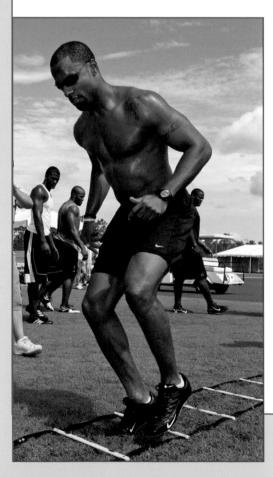

VERTIMAX

1 LUNGES

- Assume athletic stance on Vertimax platform with resistance attached to harness

- Step left foot forward to comfortable distance and lower into lunge position

until front knee is bent 90 degrees and back knee is just above ground

- Drive back into standing position by pushing through heel of left foot

- Perform set on opposite side

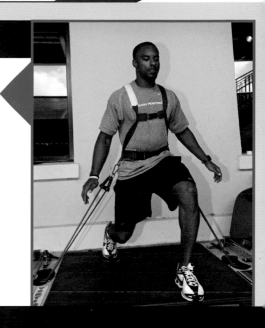

2 ANKLE FLEXOR HOPS

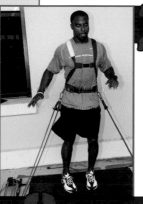

- Assume athletic stance on Vertimax platform with resistance attached to harness

- With only slight knee bend, continuously bounce on balls of feet, not allowing heels to touch ground

3 JUMP FOR HEIGHT WITH RELOAD

- Assume shoulder-width stance on Vertimax platform with resistance attached to harness

- Lower into quarter-squat, then explode straight up for maximum height

- Land softly; reset feet to shoulder width; jump again

COACHING POINTS

➤ Land softly and set your feet

➤ Keep feet shoulder-width apart and nose over toes

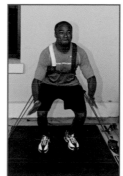

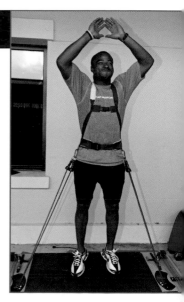

4 SHORT JUMP, HIGH JUMP

• Assume athletic stance on Vertimax platform with resistance attached to harness

• Perform quick, short hop

• Upon landing, immediately explode up for maximum height

• Repeat sequence in alternating fashion for specified reps

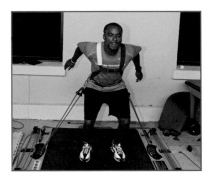

COACHING POINTS

➡ **Keep feet shoulder-width apart and nose over toes**

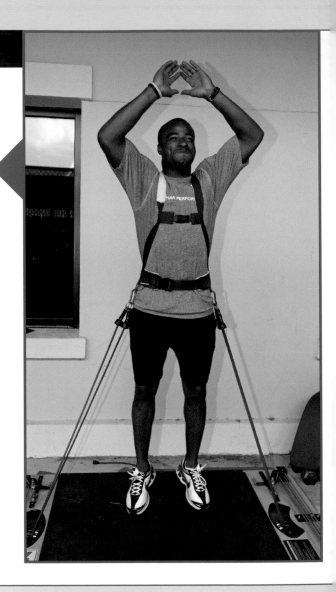

5 SPRINT

• Assume athletic stance on Vertimax platform with resistance attached to harness

• Create forward body lean against resistance and continuously simulate sprinting motion keeping toes, heels, and knees up

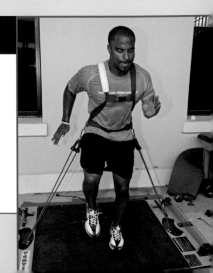

6 SINGLE-LEG JUMPS

- Assume athletic stance on Vertimax platform with resistance attached to harness

- Step forward with left foot, then explode up for maximum height off left leg

- Land softly with both legs

- Step back to start position; repeat with right leg

- Continue in alternating fashion for specified reps

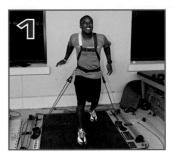
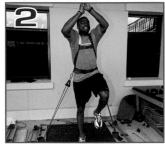
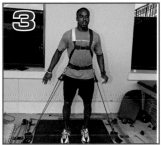

7 BOB AND WEAVE

- Assume semi-squat position on Vertimax platform with resistance attached to harness

- Keeping chest up, squat down and left as if dipping under imaginary rope

- Rise into semi-squat; repeat movement to right

- Continue bobbing and weaving for specified reps

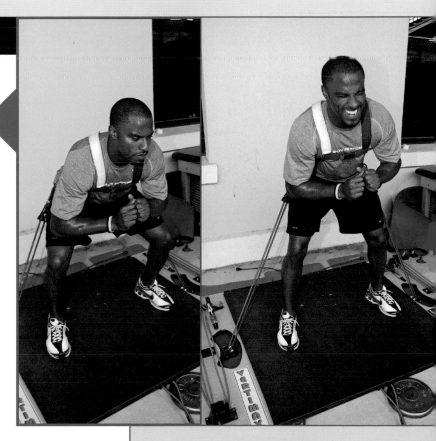

BUNGEE

STRAIGHT-AHEAD RUN

- With cord around your waist and partner holding it from behind with adequate resistance, explode off line while maintaining slight forward lean

- Partner should follow you, maintaining same cord length and resistance throughout sprint

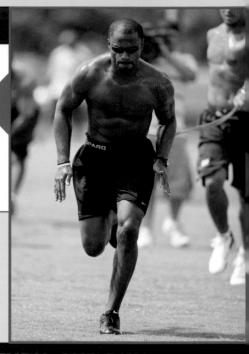

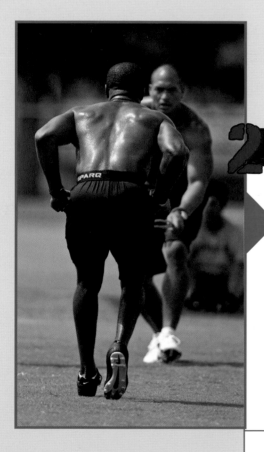

BACKPEDAL, TURN, AND RUN

- With partner holding cord in front of you, begin backpedaling

- After five yards, turn left and begin sprinting

- On next rep, turn right

COACHING POINTS

➥ Stay low throughout entire movement

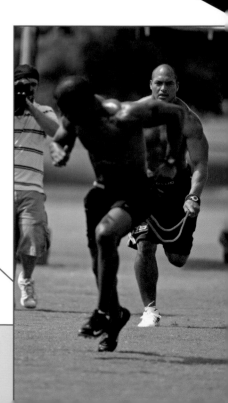

3 BACKPEDAL, BREAK ON A POST, AND SPEED TURN

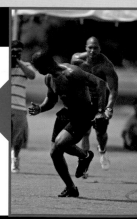

- With partner holding cord in front of you, begin backpedaling

- After five yards, break on post to left and sprint

- After another five yards, complete speed turn and sprint right

- Perform next rep on opposite side

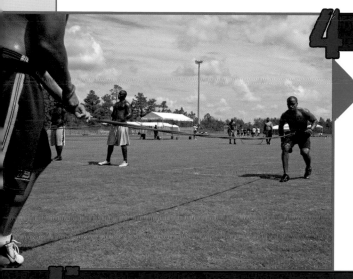

4 BACKPEDAL, BREAK FORWARD

- With partner holding cord in front of you, begin backpedaling

- After five yards, break to front and right; sprint five yards

- Cut again, then backpedal again

- After five more yards, break to front and left.

5 BACKPEDAL, BREAK, BACKPEDAL, BREAK

- Assume athletic stance in front of coach with partner providing resistance from right

- When coach points straight ahead, begin backpedaling

- React to coach's cue of pointing to his right by planting, then breaking forward and left 45 degrees

- React to coach's cue of pointing straight ahead by backpedaling

- React to coach's cue of pointing to his right by planting, then breaking forward and left 45 degrees

- Return to start; repeat for specified reps

- Perform drill breaking to right with resistance from left

Benefits: Helps you measure reaction time and build explosion

STRENGTH

BACK SQUAT

- Assume athletic stance with feet slightly wider than hip width and bar on back

- Keeping chest up, core tight and knees behind toes, lower into squat until tops of thighs are parallel to ground

- Drive up, out of squat

- Repeat for specified reps

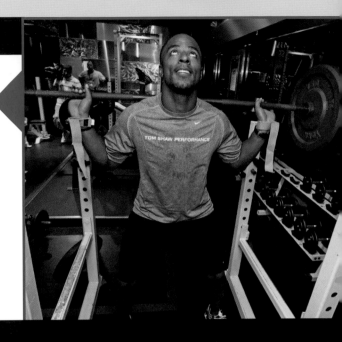

HANG CLEAN

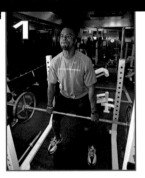
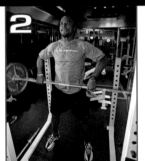
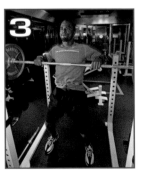
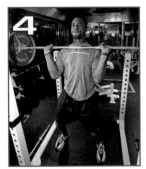

- Assume athletic stance and grasp bar with grip slightly wider than shoulder width

- Begin with bar just above knees with back locked, shoulders up, and abs and chest flexed

- Explode up by forcefully shrugging with straight arms and fully extending hips, knees and ankles

- Pull bar up, keeping it close to chest

- Drop under bar and catch it along front of shoulders in athletic stance with knees bent

- Return to start position; repeat for specified reps

COACHING POINTS

➡ Keep back arched, knees slightly bent, hips back, elbows rotated out, and shoulders up and over bar

SEATED SINGLE-LEG HAMSTRING CURL

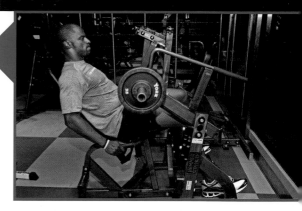

- Assume position on seated hamstring curl machine

- Contract hamstring to bring heel toward butt

- Return leg to start position with control

- Repeat for specified reps

- Perform set with opposite leg

COACHING POINTS

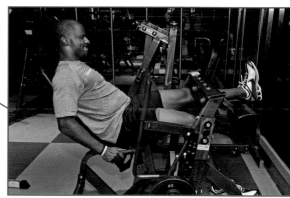

➡ Perform entire movement in slow, controlled manner

➡ Avoid squeezing or straining hamstring

➡ Do not overload weight; find comfortable starting weight

➡ Always use full extension and contraction

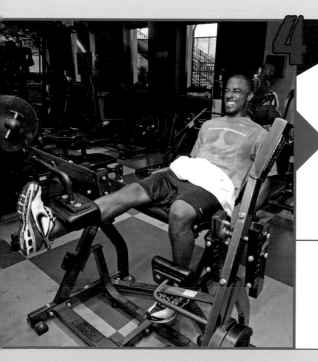

SEATED SINGLE-LEG EXTENSION

- Assume position on seated leg extension machine

- Raise weight until leg is fully extended

- Lower weight with control until knee is bent almost 90 degrees

COACHING POINTS

➡ Go through full range of motion

➡ Perform entire movement in slow, controlled manner

➡ Avoid using body to gain momentum

REAR FOOT-ELEVATED SPLIT SQUAT

Exercise can be performed holding dumbbells with foot elevated on box or bench

- On plate-loaded shrug machine, assume split-stance position

- Place back foot on shrug machine with weight on toes

- Gripping handles of shrug machine with arms at sides, lower body into squat until front knee is bent 90 degrees

- Repeat with opposite leg

COACHING POINTS

➡ When lowering into squat position, keep weight on heel of front foot, core tight, front knee behind toes, back straight, and chest high and wide

➡ Use standard squat technique with erect torso

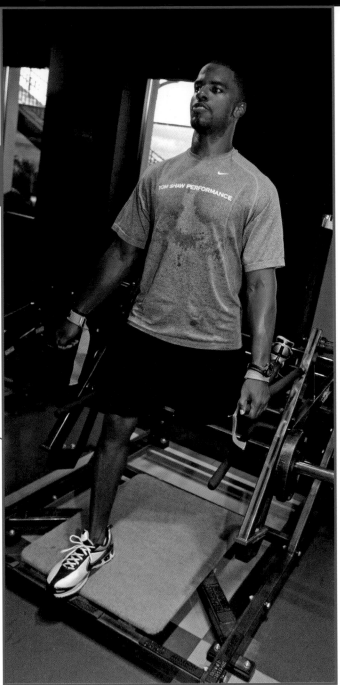

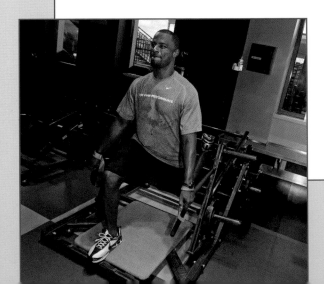

DARREN SHARPER'S TRAINING GUIDE

QUICK FEET LADDER DRILLS
Perform these drills on a track before doing them on grass.

	SETS	REST
In, Behind, Out	2-3	Walk back to start
Straight-Ahead Sprint	2-3	Walk back to start
Ricardo Coakleys	2-3	Walk back to start

VERTIMAX

	SETS/REPS
Lunges	1 X 10 each leg
Ankle Flexor Hops	1 X 10
Jump for Height With Reload	1 X 10
Short Jump, High Jump	1 X 10
Sprint	1 X 10
Single-Leg Jumps	1 X 10 each leg
Bob and Weave	1 X 10 each side

BUNGEE

	SETS	DISTANCE	REST
Straight-Ahead Run	2 with bungee, 1 without	20 yards	2 minutes
Backpedal, Turn, and Run	2 with bungee, 1 without	20 yards	2 minutes
Backpedal, Break on a Post, and Speed Turn	2 with bungee, 1 without	20 yards	2 minutes
Backpedal, Break Forward	2 with bungee, 1 without	20 yards	2 minutes
Backpedal, Break, Backpedal, Break	2 with bungee, 1 without	20 yards	2 minutes

STRENGTH

	SETS	REPS
Back Squat	3-4	10 to 12
Hang Clean	3-4	5
Seated Single-Leg Hamstring Curl	3	8
Seated Single-Leg Extension	3	8
Rear-Foot-Elevated Split Squat	3	6 each leg

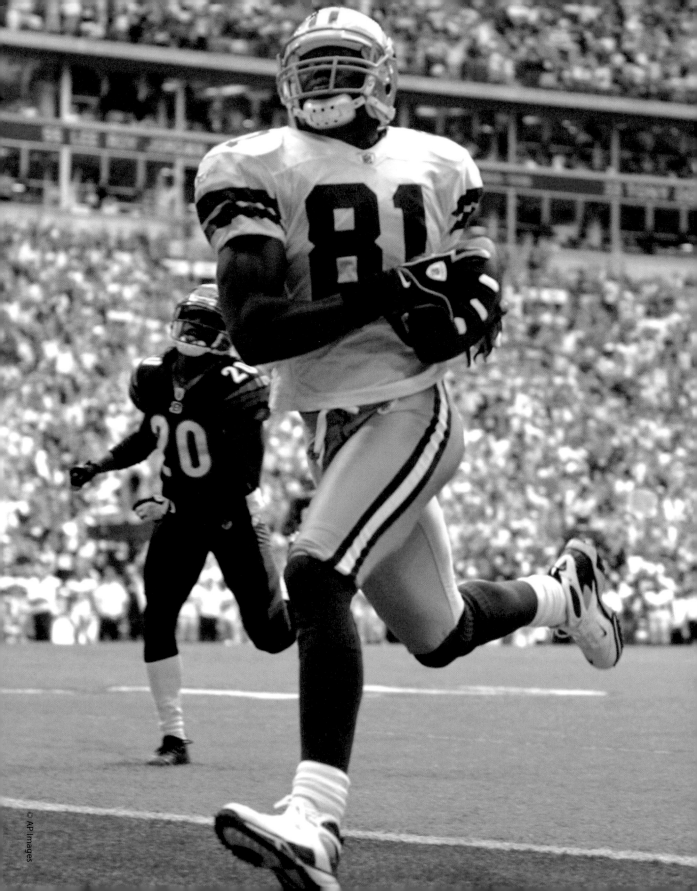

CHAPTER 2

TERRELL OWENS

EDITOR'S NOTE

Terrell Owens is undoubtedly *STACK* Magazine's most controversial cover athlete. In the summer of 2008, when the opportunity arose to highlight his off-season training program, we thought seriously about whether we could overlook all the negative attention directed at the electrifying wideout.

Our main concern was that Owens' overexposed reputation for making questionable comments and performing penalty-provoking end zone celebrations would overshadow his more positive characteristics and the tremendous story of how he reached NFL stardom. We knew that few people were aware that Owens had been a late bloomer and had worked his way through small-college football before getting noticed by NFL scouts. Or that, arguably, he continues to outwork every other player in the league. Owens is one of the few athletes who was willing and physically able to go toe-to-toe with Jerry Rice during his legendary training sessions. In fact, many of his fellow NFL players have tried to hang with Owens' current workouts and strict eating regimen, but no one has yet succeeded.

TERRELL OWENS CRUISES INTO THE END ZONE FOR A 57-YARD TOUCHDOWN AGAINST THE BENGALS IN 2008. OWENS' SPEED AND STRENGTH TRAINING HAVE MADE HIM A TOP RECEIVER IN THE NFL.

Ultimately, our decision to put Owens on the cover was based on a desire to show the little-known good side of a man who had been vilified by media and fans. We also felt that Owens was an expert in performance training and could greatly help any young athlete who was willing to sustain a high level of effort and dedication.

We spent an entire afternoon getting to know Owens at his high-rise condo in downtown Dallas. At no point during the training shoot, cover shoot, or lengthy interview did he do or say anything impolite, arrogant, or controversial. Smiling the entire time, he was extremely committed to getting his training tips and advice out to other athletes.

Despite the fact that Owens has been sent packing by Cowboys management and has signed with the Buffalo Bills, he still takes care of business on and off the field. He didn't tally his usual epic numbers during the 2008 season, but Owens has still hauled in more receiving TDs over the past three seasons [38] than any player in the league. So we stand by our decision to put Owens on our cover; we remain huge fans; and we will continue to look to him for top-of-the-line training information and inspirational content.

This is the Terrell Owens cover feature, which appeared in the October 2008 issue of *STACK* Magazine.

THE UNCOVERED RECEIVER

It's truly a shame that most of what we know about Terrell Owens comes from sensationalized stories by overzealous reporters who are more concerned with what he said into a microphone after a game than his ability to tear through defensive backs while playing it. We have heard long diatribes about the dance Owens did after scoring a particular touchdown, but not about the dedication that went into making that play possible in the first place. Overlooked is the fact that Terrell Owens is loved by his teammates and coaches and recognized as one of the hardest working and most athletic players in the game of football today.

Even the most dedicated football fans know little of Terrell Owens' story. It's about an unexceptional young athlete who found a passion, then created his own destiny around it.

While playing for his junior high football team, Owens was more likely to win a local Michael Jackson contest [yes, that really happened] than to make a play on the field. "I had just enough ability to make the team," he says. And even though he began to stand out in his last two years of high school, Owens wasn't the team's star; he didn't even crack the starting lineup until his senior year.

During those early years of athletic anonymity, a crucial catalyst in the creation of the Pro Bowl receiver we know today was formed. "During my junior and senior years, we had enrichment periods where you could study or do whatever you wanted," Owens says. "So I asked the teacher if I could get a pass to go down and lift weights. … If I didn't have any extra work to do, I was in the weight room. I was probably 6'1", 175 pounds—soaking wet. I was a stickpin, so it took a lot of hard work, dedication, and hours in that weight room."

Despite his newfound dedication, Owens' late athletic development prevented him from being a top recruit. It wasn't until the University of Tennessee–Chattanooga was recruiting one of Owens' teammates that he was noticed. "They were watching film on him," Owens recalls. "They saw a few plays I made … [and] they invited me, sort of like a package deal. I just saw my time at the University of Tennessee–Chattanooga as a means of getting an education; my mom wouldn't have been able to afford it for me."

By the time Owens got to UTC, what had started as something to do during free periods had become a deeply ingrained habit. While most of his fellow students and athletes were asleep or living up their college experiences in dorm rooms, frat houses, and common rooms around campus, Owens was honing his craft. On any given night in the off-season, any of the 8,000-plus undergrads might have noticed a fast-moving shadowy figure outside their windows. "In college, in the middle of the night, I would jump rope in the middle of the road or run sprints," Owens says. "I'm very competitive; [so] once you get those competitive juices and you want to be the best … you go the distance with it."

Reinforcing his after-hours dedication, Owens benefited from being a multi-sport collegiate athlete. He took to the hardwood as a member of the basketball team, which qualified for the 1995 NCAA tourney, and he anchored the 4x100 relay on the track team. According to Owens, the form and technique he learned running track, and the hand-eye coordination, agility, conditioning, and footwork he developed playing basketball helped him take his football game to a higher level. Owens, who eventually hit 6'3" and more than 200 pounds, developed into a fast, coordinated receiver. And despite being keyed on and double-covered almost his entire senior season, he posted numbers that NFL scouts couldn't overlook.

In 1996, when the San Francisco 49ers drafted Owens in the third round, he got his chance to play in the NFL. "I can't say that it's always been a dream," Owens says. "It's just

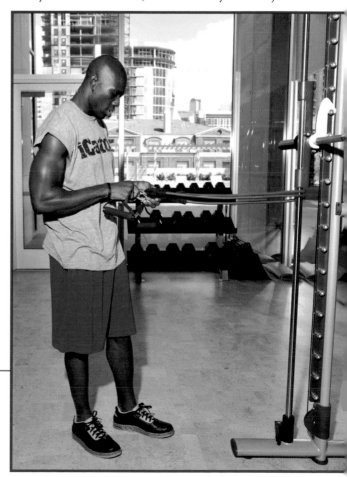

something that I've always been competitive with. I think a lot of guys giving interviews or in a spur of the moment will say, 'I've always dreamed of this moment.' God blessed me with a lot of talent and a lot of ability, and it was something that I tapped into and honed my skills and tried to perfect the craft. As I've matured and learned to play the game of football, the dream for me is to win a championship—and that's what I strive to do each and every year."

Since entering the NFL, Owens has continued to mature and perfect his craft, getting hungrier each year. "I learned from the best in the game at my position—Jerry Rice," he says. "I knew that I had to prepare every off-season like I was the number-one guy. I wanted to be the playmaker, the go-to guy. In the fourth quarter, you want to be the guy that can be counted on in those crunch seconds of a game. I want to be a guy my teammates depend on.

"When I prepare myself for each season," he continues, "those are the things that go through my mind. It's all about having that love and passion for the game. I don't think anyone can ever dispute that I have that passion for the game or [that I] go out there and display it every weekend."

Shredded Up To Pieces

In the middle of performing his intense—almost obsessive—strength training routine, Owens sums up his approach in one neat package. While patting his chest, shoulders and arms, he says: "These are my babies. I have to keep them strong." He then holds out his open hands in front of him: "And these are my moneymakers!"

For Owens, owning the NFL's best physique and the most effective moves off the line is no accident. A realization early in his career fueled the development of both. "In my third year in the league, I was introduced to a trainer who I currently have, Buddy Primm," Owens says. "Once I got with him, I realized how bad of shape I was in—even when I thought I was in good shape."

Following this discovery, Owens set out on a journey to get into the best shape possible and to educate himself on what was most beneficial for his game. As a result, his training methods changed drastically. "When you don't have the knowledge, you go through junior high, high school, and college … all about impressing the girls—how much you bench press, how much can you curl, how much you can squat," he says. "That is the traditional stuff that everyone learned growing up. But once you become knowledgeable about your body and what you are trying to obtain with it, you start to get into innovative and creative stuff. Once I got away from that traditional stuff and starting doing my own thing, I saw a big difference in my body make-up."

Owens' search for the innovative and creative brought him to elastic band training. "I injured my groin and did some work with a guy who used bands to strengthen those muscles," Owens recalls. "I could just feel it strengthening me from the inside. And most people don't know this, but a lot of your speed comes from your core, inside out. From that point on, I wanted to incorporate bands into my training."

So impressed with the results was Owens that he teamed up with Bodylastics to create the T.O. Strongman Edition training bands, which support heavy-duty strength training at a higher resistance than traditional bands.

With this system, Owens has created an upper-body workout suited to the demands of the wide receiver position. "I do a lot of work with my hands coming off the line [to] prevent a DB from jamming me up or getting off with different releases," he says. "If I have a defender in front of me, I have my hands up and in front the whole time on the line. Depending on his body position, I'm either going to rip through, swim through, or catch him off guard and drive my hands straight into him at the same time. That's why I do a lot band work that isolates the muscles in each hand, because everything I do is with one arm or one hand."

Owens' training re-education came with a new approach to nutrition—a combination that's produced exponential results. "My first couple years, I was eating McDonalds, Pizza Hut, Domino's, and Burger King. I had to weed all that stuff out," he says. "[Buddy] introduced healthy eating and [the idea of] eating every

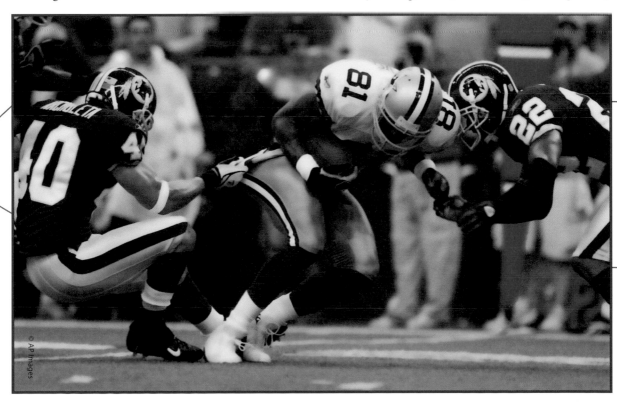

© AP Images

three to four hours throughout the day—at least four to five meals a day, [which is] to speed your metabolism up."

Owens now eats eight to 10 egg whites and oatmeal in the morning. If he happens to hit up the Waffle House, he'll order steamed hash browns, and when he wants chocolate, he'll snack on veggies instead. "It's crazy sometimes and gets monotonous. Many people have tried to stick to my diet, and they can't do it," he says. "But this on top of the training, it's going to shred you up to pieces."

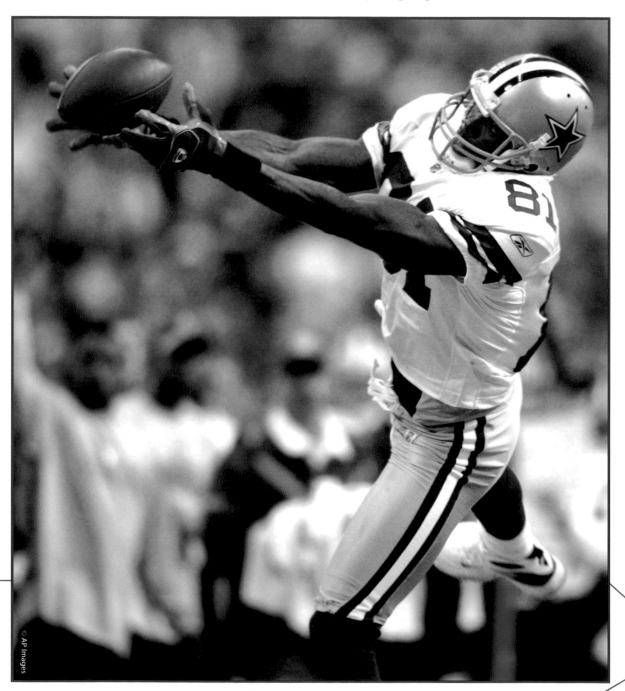

© AP Images

BAND TRAINING

CHEST PRESS

Owens: You can rep out with this just like a 225 Combine sort of thing.
Just rep out until you feel the burn.

- With band resistance attached to stable object behind you, step forward into staggered stance holding handles at chest level

- Drive handles straight ahead by fully extending arms

- Return arms to start position with control; repeat for specified reps

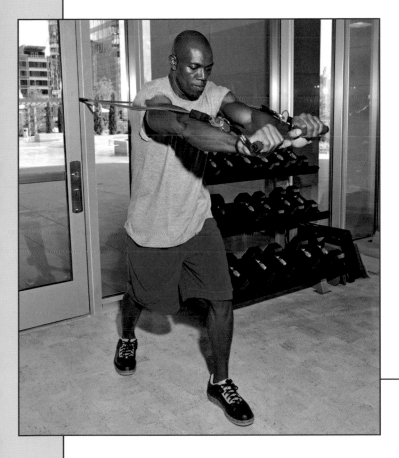

COACHING POINTS

- ➤ Keep core tight
- ➤ Get into position with sound base
- ➤ Push straight ahead, just like bench press

2 SEATED ROW

Owens: You'll feel this in your back and the tops of your shoulders. This helps so much with muscle balance and being able to take and deliver a blow. It gives you all that power behind you when you're trying to deliver a blow. You can increase the resistance by adding bands, or you can move yourself back to increase the tension.

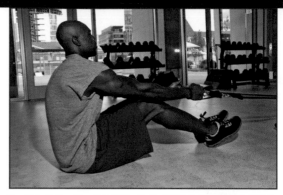

- With band resistance attached to stable object at low position in front, sit on ground holding handles with arms straight forward

- Drive elbows back until hands reach chest

- Return arms to start position with control; repeat for specified reps

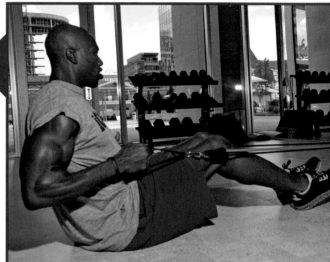

Coaching Points

➡ Keep upper body straight
➡ Stay stationary
➡ Let arms do the work; don't rock

3 SHOULDER PRESS

Owens: This is good for the traps and shoulders. I crouch down a little to get myself a good base, so I'm not wobbly—and I'm tightening my abs. I have a technique now that my trainer gave me; he tells me to "key up." It's kind of like if you have to go to the bathroom and you cut it off; that's what I'm doing the whole time— and [I] make sure my butt isn't sticking out.

- Assume athletic, staggered stance

- Hold handles at shoulder level with band under back foot

- Drive handles toward ceiling until arms are straight

- Lower with control; repeat for specified reps

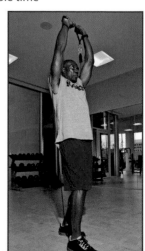

Coaching Points

➡ Establish good base ➡ Keep core tight

4 SINGLE-ARM CROSSOVER

Owens: I'm working my core and pec at the same time. Again, I don't have my butt sticking out; I'm keyed up. Start at a distance that puts some tension in the band.

• With band resistance attached to stable object to left, hold handle with left arm to side with tension in band

• Keeping body stable, bring arm across body to right

• Return arm to start position with control; repeat for specified reps

• Perform set on right side

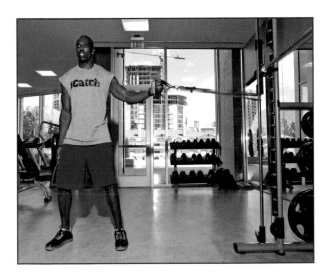

COACHING POINTS

➤ Keep core tight
➤ Bring arm to middle and across chest
➤ Feel isolation in chest

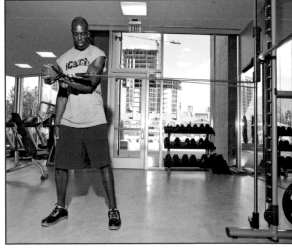

Owens: You'll really feel this in the back and across your shoulders. You can do these with dumbbells, but I like to use the bands, because they're easier on the joints; the movement is much more fluid, and it's constant resistance. The more you spread your feet, the harder it is, because it's more tension. This strengthens the shoulders and all the smaller intrinsic muscles on the inside. In football, there are a lot of guys with shoulder problems, because you can get hit every kind of way; you can have an awkward fall; you can get hit on your shoulder. The stronger those internal muscles are, the better your chances of healing and coming back faster.

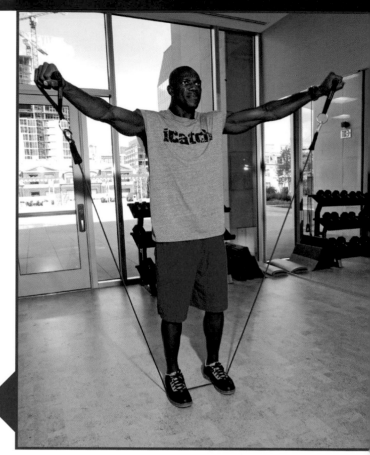

- Assume athletic stance with band under feet; hold handles at sides with arms angled slightly forward

- Keeping arms straight, raise them to shoulder level and slightly in front

- Lower arms to start position; repeat for specified reps

COACHING POINTS

➡ **Keep eyes focused straight ahead**

➡ **Do not use body to create momentum**

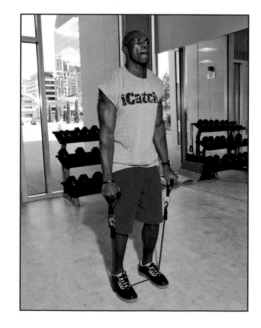

FRONT RAISE

Owens: You can feel your shoulders burn all up the front; you get a different burn from the different angle.

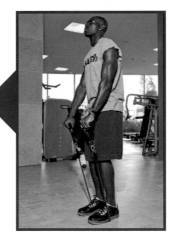

- Assume athletic stance with band under feet; hold handles in front of thighs with palms facing you

- Keeping arms straight, raise them to shoulder level in front of you

- Lower arms to start position; repeat for specified reps

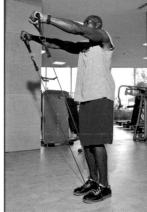

COACHING POINTS

- ➤ Keep feet shoulder-width apart
- ➤ Focus on driving straight up with arms
- ➤ Keep tension on band when you come back down

REAR DELT

- With band resistance attached to stable object in front, step back into even stance; hold handles with arms straight in front of you and tension in band

- Keeping arms straight, bring handles back and to side until they are even with shoulders

- Return arms to start position with control; repeat for specified reps

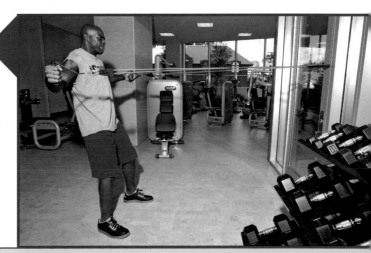

Owens: This is a traditional curl. A lot of people use dumbbells, but with these bands you get resistance on the way up and on the way down. You get a constant pump.

• Assume athletic stance with band under feet; hold handles in front of thighs with palms facing out

• Without changing position of elbows, bring handles to chest level by curling arms

• Return arms to start position with control; repeat for specified reps

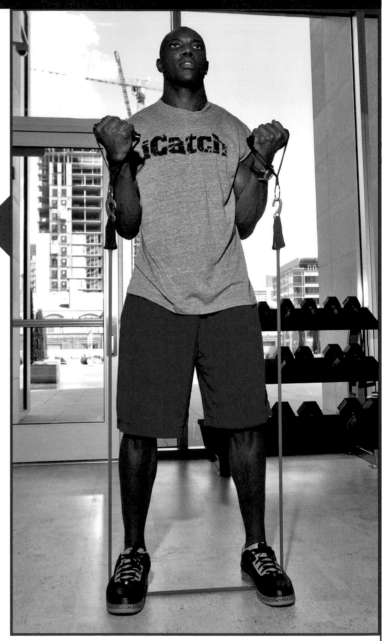

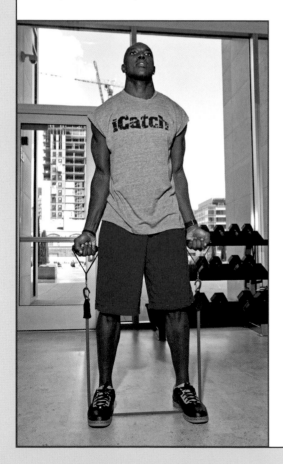

COACHING POINTS

➡ Keep arms shoulder-width apart and elbows in tight

➡ Bring arms up to just more than parallel

TERRELL OWENS' TRAINING GUIDE

BAND TRAINING

	SETS	REPS
Chest Press	4	15
Seated Row	4	15
Shoulder Press	4	13-15
Single-Arm Crossover	4	10-12
Adjusted Lateral Raise	4	13-15
Front Raise	4	13-15
Rear Delt	4	13-15
Bicep Curl	4	13-15

CHAPTER 3

PITTSBURGH STEELERS

EDITOR'S NOTE

In the fall of 2005, seven months after launching *STACK* Magazine, we received an unsolicited call from Robert Fitzpatrick, assistant strength coach for the Pittsburgh Steelers and one of *Men's Journal*'s Top 100 Trainers in America. As soon as Fitzpatrick heard about *STACK*, he became interested in contributing, particularly about his innovative speed training, which focuses heavily on reaction.

A month after our initial phone call, we were on the road to Pittsburgh to work with Fitzpatrick and attend one of the Steelers' post-practice speed sessions.

Tennis balls, surprisingly, were Fitzpatrick's training tool of choice when working with these gridiron greats, and he used them liberally in his drills. A Who's Who of superstars participated, including Hines Ward, Ike Taylor, and Deshea Townsend. Also participating was a little-known linebacker from Kent State University—James Harrison. Three years after our shoot, Harrison set a Steelers record for sacks in a season, becoming the NFL's Defensive Player of the Year.

JAMES HARRISON SETS OFF ON A 100-YARD INTERCEPTION RETURN IN THE PITTSBURGH STEELERS' 2009 SUPER BOWL VICTORY OVER THE ARIZONA CARDINALS. SPEED WORKOUTS HELPED HARRISON OUTRUN THE CARDINALS IN PURSUIT ON THE PLAY.

The article featuring this speed workout appeared in our February 2006 issue. That month marked not only our company's first anniversary, but also the Steelers' *fifth* Super Bowl championship. Any workout that can improve the attributes of the Steelers' already-gifted roster and lead to championships, is fame-worthy and deserving of a spot in our top 10 favorite football workouts.

A year after the Steelers' 2006 title victory, head coach Bill Cowher retired. Fitzpatrick followed Cowher in exiting the team, but he continues to work independently with athletes of all levels, helping them improve their athleticism, speed and reaction. And although Fitzgerald has separated from the Steelers, it's a safe bet that his workouts from 2004 to 2006 contributed to their Super Bowl title in 2009—No. 6 for the franchise.

MIND GAMES

Pittsburgh Steelers speed coach Robert Fitzpatrick shares a mental twist that will help you take your game to the next level.

When the Pittsburgh Steelers went from 6–10 in 2003 to 15–1 in 2004, people couldn't help but ask, "What did these guys do after the 2003 season?"

Yeah, picking up Pro Bowl running back Duce Staley from the Philadelphia Eagles helped. And who can deny the impact of 2004 first-round draft pick, "Big Ben" Roethlisberger? The young QB from Miami of Ohio didn't lose a regular-season game until his 16th pro start.

However, major acquisitions were not limited to the field. The Steelers also hired assistant strength coach Robert Fitzpatrick. The two-time selection as one of *Men's Journal's* Top 100 Trainers in America flipped the team's program on its head.

On his first day, Fitzpatrick asked each player what part of his game he wanted to enhance. "A lot of the guys said explosiveness and first-step speed. From their answers, I produced a program based on explosive movements and plyometric drills," he says. "But what makes this program really different is that it challenges them as much mentally as it does physically."

Fitzpatrick refers to his mental training as "the next level." He says that when two athletes of equal size, strength, and speed go head-to-head, the one who can maintain mental focus longer will win.

The drills Fitzpatrick uses develop first-step explosiveness and reaction time while also challenging the athlete mentally. His technique involves nothing more than a tennis ball or the opening and closing of his fist.

"I use tennis balls and other visual cues with every drill," he explains. "The athlete can't start a rep until I drop the tennis ball or open or close my fist. This way, he's always thinking, staying focused on the ball or my hand, and then reacting as fast as possible to perform an explosive movement. The combination of cue and movement incorporates the dynamics of football into my training. Every play is based on reacting to something you see. Your first step then has to be fast and explosive."

The Steelers perform the following five drills [among many other essential speed-training drills] twice a week in the off-season. "The guys love these drills because they are challenging; they love being tested," Fitzpatrick says. "And the drills have greatly improved their first-step quickness, which is crucial to every position on the field, from corner to linebacker to lineman."

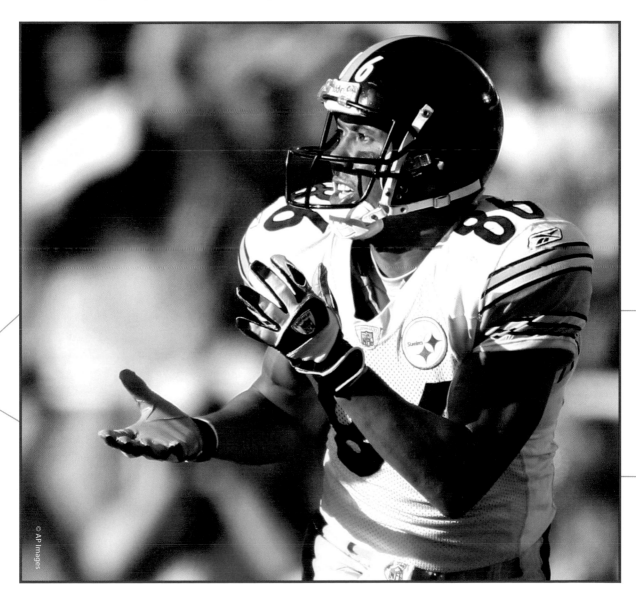

© AP Images

HINES WARD HAULS IN A PASS DURING A GAME IN 2006. WARD'S CONDITIONING HAS HELPED HIM TO ENJOY A LONG NFL CAREER.

EXPLOSIVE REACTION TRAINING

EXPLOSIVE PRONE REACTION STARTS

- Assume push-up position with partner five yards in front with tennis ball in each hand

- Designate which of partner's hands is "reaction hand" and which of your legs is "drive leg"

- When partner drops ball from reaction hand, explode forward into sprint by bringing designated leg underneath and driving out

- Repeat for specified reps, alternating drive leg and partner's reaction hand

Benefits: Increases mental focus // Explosive first steps // Reaction time

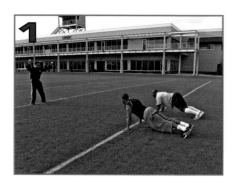

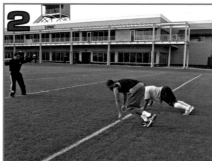

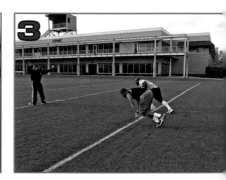

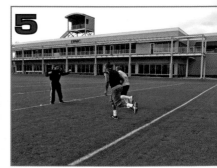

COACHING POINTS

➡ Do not catch tennis ball because of the torque it puts on knees

EXPLOSIVE PLYO REACTION BOUNDS

- Stand with right foot on 18-inch plyo box with partner holding tennis ball in front of you

- When partner drops ball, react by driving through box with right leg to explode straight up

- Drive left knee and right arm up to achieve maximum height

- Land in starting position; repeat for specified reps as partner drops ball

- Perform set with left leg on box

Benefits: Increases explosive power and acceleration // Develops proper drive angles

COACHING POINTS

➡ Focus on speed of reaction and explosiveness of movement off box

➡ Avoid emphasizing how fast you land, and get back into starting position after jump

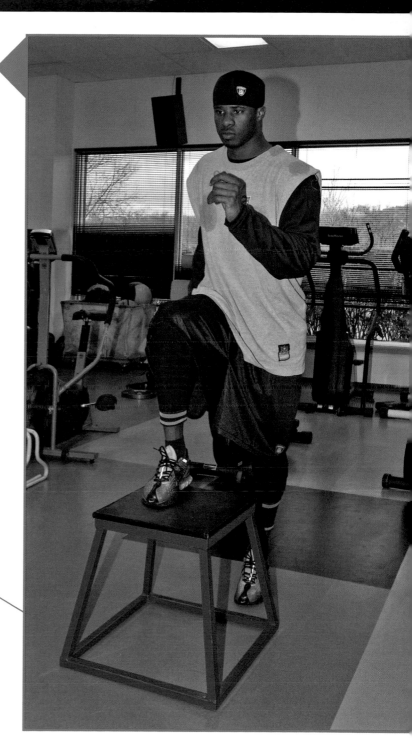

HV JUMP

- Assume staggered stance behind mini hurdle with 18-inch plyo box few feet in front

- React to partner's ball drop by jumping off both feet over mini hurdle

- Land softly between mini hurdle and box, then immediately jump onto box

- Land softly on box, step down and return to start position

- Repeat for specified reps

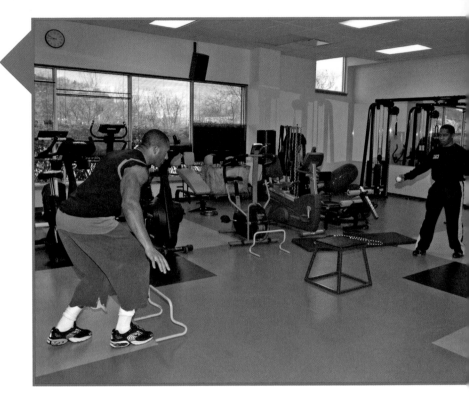

Benefits: Increases game speed and reaction time

EXPLOSIVE LATERAL BOX STEPS

• Stand to left of 18-inch plyo box and mini hurdle with partner holding tennis ball in front

• When partner drops ball, react by quickly stepping right foot laterally over mini hurdle and onto box

• Step left foot onto box

• Step down into start position; repeat for specified reps as partner drops ball

Benefits: Enhances lateral quickness // Develops back leg strength and explosion

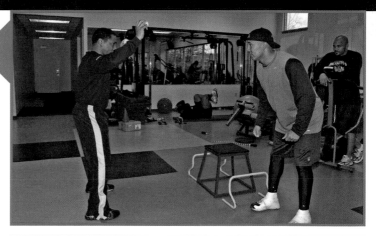

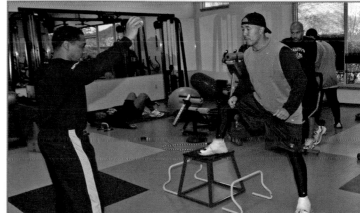

COACHING POINTS

➥ Perform with staggered stance to incorporate football dynamics

➥ Avoid training with your feet square, because it does not mimic on-field football movements

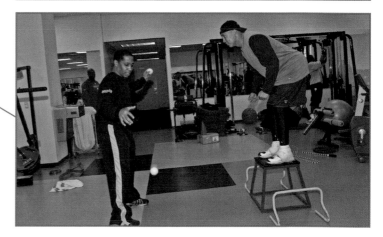

FIRST-STEP FOCUS DRILL

Set up four cones in a square, each side being 10 yards long. Number cones 1 through 4, counterclockwise.

• Assume athletic stance in center of square

• Sprint to Cone 1, plant and backpedal to center

• Shuffle to Cone 2, shuffle back to center

• Shuffle to Cone 4, shuffle back to center

• Backpedal to Cone 3, plant and sprint to center

Adaptation: Have partner stand near Cone 1 and hold up finger(s) indicating which cone to move to // Follow visual commands for 20 seconds

Benefits: Sharpens mental focus // Increases change-of-direction speed // Enhances ability to stop, start and pivot // Develops reaction time based on visual cues

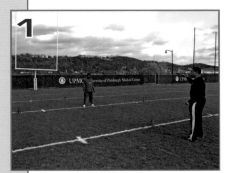

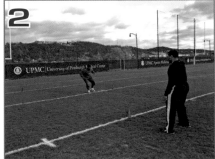

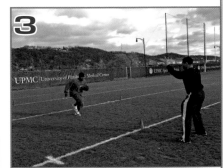

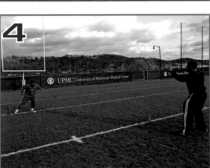

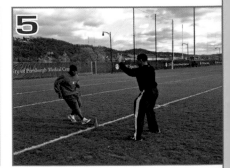

STEELERS TRAINING GUIDE

EXPLOSIVE REACTION TRAINING

	SETS	REPS	REST
Explosive Prone Reaction Starts	1	5 each leg	
Explosive Plyo Reaction Bounds	6	8x6	15 seconds between reps
HV Jump	8	10	
Explosive Lateral Box Steps	8	10 each direction	
First-Step Focus Drill	1	4-6	40-60 seconds between sets

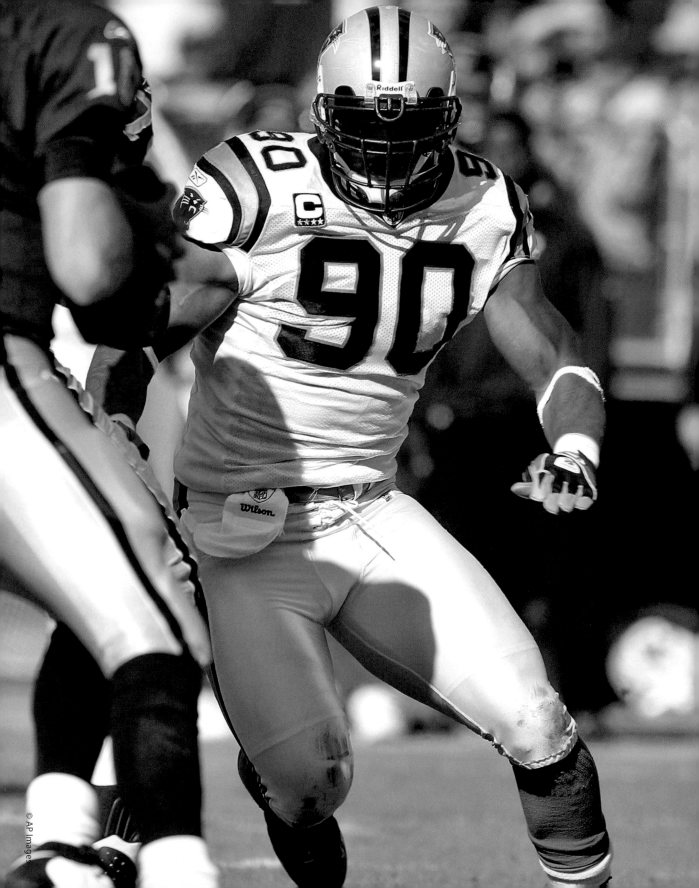

CHAPTER 4

JULIUS PEPPERS

EDITOR'S NOTE

Watching a 6′7″, 285-pound man move in a coordinated, fluid, and explosive manner can be frightening—which is exactly how we felt when we saw Julius Peppers perform an off-season workout with Danny Arnold, owner of Plex in Stafford, Texas. The pair agreed to have us down during the summer of 2005, right after Peppers' historic 2004 season, during which he made countless tackles and racked up 11 sacks. We took advantage of the opportunity to witness and report the training of one of the world's best two-sport athletes [Peppers worked the hardwood as well as the gridiron as a student-athlete at the University of North Carolina].

Judging by Peppers' large, defined frame, we assumed that his training involved a lot of heavy weights. We soon learned that Peppers didn't meddle with the metal; instead, he focused on fast, athletic, football-specific movements. In fact, Peppers told us that he felt lifting weights had actually hindered his career early on, because his muscle mass had increased so drastically.

Leaving the traditional weight bar behind, Peppers proceeded to attack pretty much every moveable object in the gym, alternating between explosive sled drives and partner-resisted

JULIUS PEPPERS CLOSES IN ON THE QUARTERBACK DURING A GAME AGAINST THE RAIDERS IN 2008. PEPPERS' SIZE AND EXPLOSIVE ABILITY MAKE HIM A FORCE IN THE NFL.

exercises, which forced him to work through nearly every possible movement pattern—all of which he dominated. Few athletes have to work to keep their muscle mass in check. But training explosively with athletic movements is a wise strategy for anyone looking for an improved on-field performance. For that reason, Peppers' training ranks in our top 10 football workouts and adds a ton of value to this book.

Despite his intimidating stature, Peppers was quiet and shy when we met with him. Once he opened up, though, he was very direct about his past experiences. He related how he had veered off course at times in the past, but had since found discipline [and Arnold]. The word "Discipline" is tattooed on top of one of his wrists, the word "Dedication" on the other.

During the past couple of seasons, Peppers has continued to develop as an athlete with those two virtues in mind. In 2008, he tallied 14.5 sacks, 51 tackles and four forced fumbles while leading the Panthers into the NFL playoffs. In addition, he has continued to mature, easily assuming the role of team leader in Carolina. Peppers is now considered one of the best defensive players in the game.

The following is the cover feature on Julius Peppers from the December 2006 issue of *STACK* Magazine.

FULL GROWN

I live by two things every day—discipline and dedication—in whatever I am doing, not just football. I feel like those are the keys to life. The dedication has always been with me, but I have had to work on the discipline over the years. I wasn't always doing the right things to get to where I wanted to be. —Julius Peppers

At the age of 15, Julius Peppers stood 6'5", weighed 225 pounds, and was the fastest, most athletic student at Southern Nash Senior High School in Bailey, North Carolina. With the skill to dominate both the gridiron and hardwood, Peppers knew early on that his body would guide him to fame and fortune. However, even though he had the power and ability of a grown man, he lacked the guidance and direction necessary to succeed.

"When I was in eighth or ninth grade, I knew I'd be offered a scholarship," Peppers says. "And that's tough when you're young, because you have a lot of distractions. Once people recognize that you can be a college athlete—or maybe a pro athlete—they start pulling on you. You have to keep your circle of friends and family real tight, and keep your eyes open so you're aware of all the negative things and can distance yourself from them."

Although Peppers tried constantly, he wasn't always able to keep the distractions in check. The summer before his freshman year at the University of North Carolina, the school's dean booted Peppers from the summer orientation program for numerous curfew violations and because he used a university stipend to buy a pair of Air Jordan shoes, which were mistakenly sent to the Office of the Dean instead of then-head basketball coach Dean Smith's office. Sent packing and told not to return until classes started, Peppers had veered off course before the semester even began and marked himself as a problem child for newly hired freshman advisor Carl Carey.

During his first days at UNC, Carey, who has a Ph.D. in educational psychology, was briefed on the football star. "I first met Carl my freshman year when he was assigned as the academic advisor for the whole freshman class," Peppers says. "But it ended up that he was specifically assigned to keep me in line. I came pretty close to failing out of UNC that first year, but Carl walked me through everything and helped me get through it."

While Carey was prepping Peppers for tests and retests in courses like Drama 15, Peppers was doing just fine for himself when it came to his game. During the 2000 football season, he established himself as a top pass rusher in college football, setting a school record with 24 tackles for a loss, and coming within one sack of tying Lawrence Taylor's single-season school mark of 16 sacks. On the court, he developed into a bruising power forward, leading the Tar Heels to the Final Four in 2000. In 2001—his last season with UNC—Peppers won the Lombardi Award as the nation's top lineman and the Chuck Bednarik Award as the nation's top defensive player. These accolades solidified his position as a top 2002 NFL Draft pick.

Balancing two sports at a big-time college was at times difficult for Peppers, but he believes it benefited him in both arenas. "Basketball helped me with my footwork and gave me a much more athletic style of play in football," he says. "But the physical nature and aggressiveness of being a football player helped me bang with the big boys down low."

In 2002, when draft time rolled around for the dual-sport athlete, Carey became more than

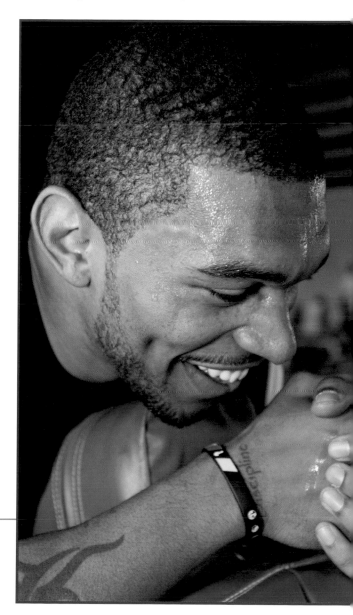

Peppers' academic advisor. Noticing the endless phone calls Peppers was getting from shady agents, Carey began screening the requests and became the talking head for the future star. Eventually, Peppers handed over all draft duties to Carey, letting him make the major decisions. Carey's help paid off; the Carolina Panthers selected Peppers as the second overall pick.

Along the way, Peppers grew up by learning from his mistakes and from the guidance of a key advisor—now his friend and agent. "I have seen a lot of guys who were as talented as me, or maybe even more talented, who didn't make it, because they didn't have the right people around them," Peppers says. "Now that I am fully grown, I know the importance of doing the right thing, and I've learned how to do it."

Since college, Peppers' growth has entailed straightening up his off-field hiccups, taking home the 2002 NFL Rookie of the Year Award and leading the Panthers to the Super Bowl in 2003. His 2004 Pro Bowl season was one of the most impressive ever by a defensive lineman, with 52 tackles, 11 sacks, two interceptions, four forced fumbles, and two touchdowns. Knowing there is still room for growth, Peppers has used his vow of dedication and discipline to leave the distractions and negative experiences behind.

Moving On

Even at his stature, Peppers can outrun receivers and overpower linemen. His rare combination of speed, size, power, and explosion makes Peppers one of the most menacing

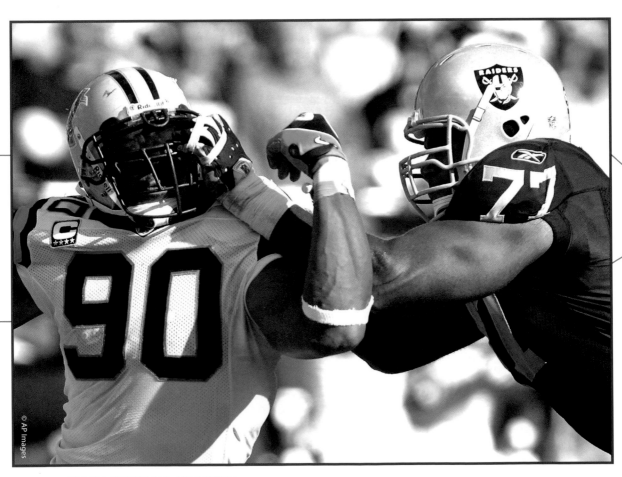

© AP Images

defenders in the game. Responsible for helping Peppers maintain his freakish ability is Danny Arnold, owner of Plex [Stafford, Texas].

Although Peppers didn't train in high school—or even warm up before games for that matter—he got pretty serious about pumping iron at UNC. "When I was in high school, I just went out and played," he says. "But when I got to college, I started lifting weights and got really big—up to 300 pounds. I was tight all over and could barely move. I was tripping over my own feet, so I knew it wasn't good for me as a football player."

When it was time to train for the 2002 NFL Draft, Carey—Peppers' right-hand man—did some research and discovered that Danny Arnold was one of the best at prepping players for the NFL Combine and their Pro Days. Following Carey's advice yet again, Peppers headed to Stafford to begin training with Arnold. To say Peppers' Pro Day was impressive is an understatement. "They laid out the long mat with numbers on it to measure his standing broad jump," Arnold explains. "Peppers lined up, then jumped all the way off the mat. Everyone just stared at each other—no one had ever seen that before."

Since blowing away the scouts at his Pro Day, Peppers has returned to Plex every off-season but one to partake in workouts that are as unusual as his athletic ability. The training has helped Peppers put his mark on the league, becoming the standard against whom all other defensive ends are measured. "Some guys like to do a lot of benching and squatting—all that powerlifting stuff," Peppers says. "But I have a style of play that is more athletic and relies on flexibility. It doesn't benefit me a whole lot being strong like that. With these workouts here, I stay loose and flexible. And Danny's training is always fresh and different, which is like playing football."

Synchronizing Peppers' training with the game of football is Arnold's main goal, and he pulls it off by designing drills that incorporate movement, explosion, and balance on the turf—where the game is played. "The power clean is a great exercise to an extent," Arnold says. "But after awhile, it just makes you better at performing the power clean. That's why I train Peppers with football-related movements—so that he gets better at them."

Arnold even keeps the environment inside Plex as football-like as possible. "When it's really hot outside, we don't shut the doors and windows and crank up the AC like your local health club does," he says. "We keep everything like it is when you play football. It gets hot and sweaty in here; sometimes it's tough to breathe."

With every year that he's returned to Plex, Peppers has continually developed and improved his already-unfair athleticism. "Danny has helped with my explosion and quick-twitch muscles throughout the whole game," he says. "I have a burst that stays with me through the third and fourth quarters. I didn't work with Danny before [the 2005] season, and I noticed how tired I was getting during the games. I didn't have that speed around the edge, so I knew I had to come back."

Although he's best known for racking up sacks, picks, fumble recoveries, and defensive TDs, Peppers is not concerned with those numbers. "Getting back to the Super Bowl is the main goal—it's what I play for," he says. "I don't set personal goals, and statistics don't hold a lot of value for me. It really doesn't bother me if I'm not in the top three leaders in sacks, as long as I am doing what I need to help my team win."

WARM-UP

Before Peppers hits the sled for his on-field workout, he first goes through a vigorous warm up routine, focusing on the hips, shoulders, and core to loosen up the joints while breaking a little sweat.

PHYSIOBALL VERTICAL RAISE

- Lie with chest on ball, holding light dumbbells in hands with thumbs pointing up

- Keeping arms straight, raise dumbbells to head level with arms in Y position and palms facing down

- Lower dumbbells to start position with control

- Repeat for specified reps

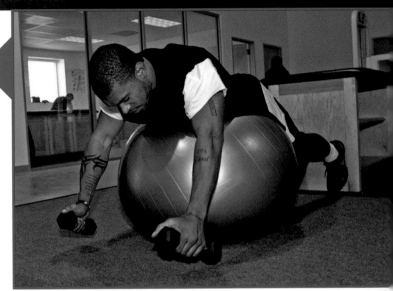

COACHING POINTS

- ➡ Focus on balancing core on ball
- ➡ Control arms going up and down
- ➡ Use light weight

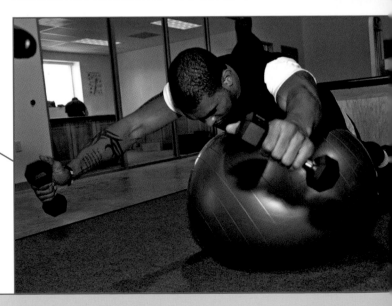

2 PHYSIOBALL PRESS

- Lie with chest on ball, holding light dumbbells at head level with arms bent 90 degrees

- Without allowing arms to drop below head level, slowly press weights straight ahead until arms are fully extended

- Return dumbbells to start position; repeat for specified reps

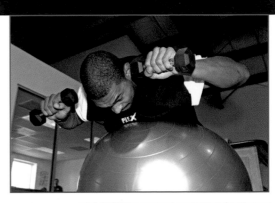

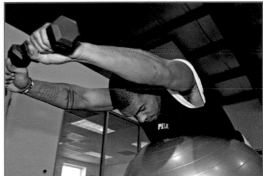

COACHING POINTS

➡ **Use light weight**
➡ **Focus on balancing core on ball**
➡ **Fully extend arms**

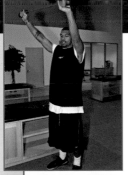

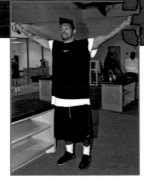

3 BAND PULL-APART

- Hold band overhead so hands are shoulder-width apart and band has tension

- Slowly pull band apart to create more tension; return to start position

- Slowly lower arms to eye level; repeat drill at eye level

- Slowly lower arms to chest level; repeat drill at chest level

- Repeat alternating motions for specified reps

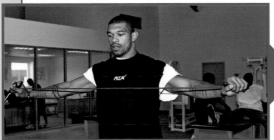

COACHING POINTS

➡ **Keep tension in band at all times**
➡ **Use slow, controlled movements**

4 SINGLE-ARM DUMBBELL EXTERNAL ROTATION

- Lying on side, hold dumbbell in upper hand with elbow bent 90 degrees

- Keeping elbow bent 90 degrees and pinned against side, externally rotate shoulder to bring dumbbell parallel to body

- Lower dumbbell with control to start position through same movement pattern

- Repeat for specified reps; perform set with opposite arm

COACHING POINTS

➡ **Use light weight**
➡ **Keep elbow bent 90 degrees**
➡ **Use shoulder, not arm, to rotate**

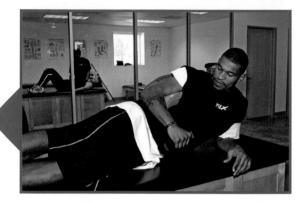

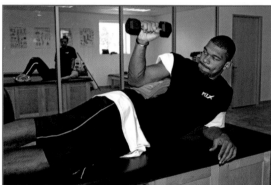

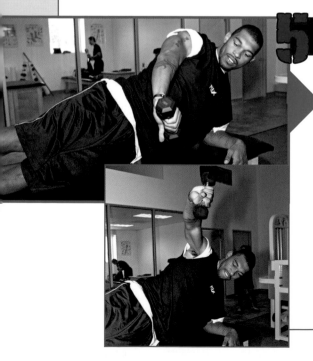

5 SINGLE-ARM SIDE DUMBBELL RAISE

- Lying on side, hold light dumbbell with arm extended and rotated so that pinky finger is toward ceiling

- Leading with pinky finger, raise arm as high as range of motion allows

- Lower arm with control to start position; repeat for specified reps

- Perform set with opposite arm

COACHING POINTS

➡ **Use light weight** ➡ **Keep arm straight** ➡ **Move slowly**

OPPOSITE HAND TOE TOUCH

- Standing on one foot on stability pad, hold light med ball in hand opposite balancing leg

- Keeping arm extended and balancing leg straight, simultaneously rotate and bend at waist to bring med ball down toward balancing foot

- Return to start position through same movement pattern; repeat for specified reps

- Perform set on opposite leg

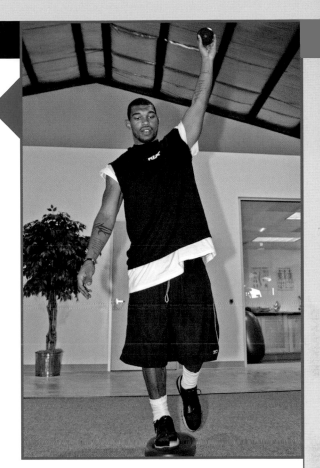

COACHING POINTS

- ➡ Keep leg and arm straight
- ➡ Focus on staying balanced
- ➡ Rotate at hip, not shoulder

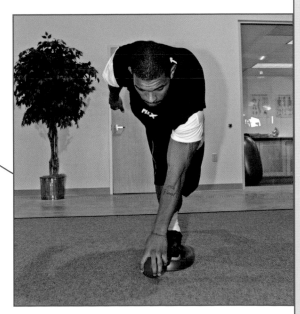

SINGLE-ARM SHOULDER BALANCE

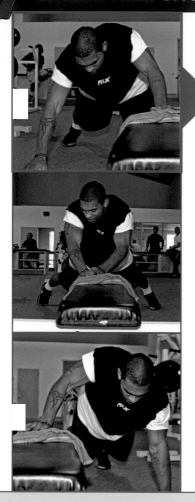

- Assume push-up position on ground with bench to left

- Step left hand up onto bench while stabilizing with right shoulder

- Bring right hand up onto bench

- Step left hand down onto ground left of bench

- Step right hand down to ground to assume push-up position

- Repeat sequence in opposite direction

- Continue for specified reps

COACHING POINTS

➡ **Keep back flat**
➡ **Focus on controlling body balance**
➡ **Keep head facing floor**

BASKETBALL WALL DRIBBLE

- Balance on right leg, holding basketball overhead with right hand

- Dribble ball on wall for set duration; switch sides

COACHING POINTS

➡ **Focus on balance** ➡ **Reach as high as possible**
➡ **Use fingertips to dribble ball**

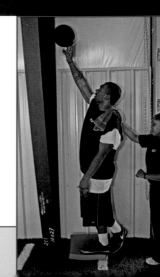

FIELD WORK

Arnold, who believes strongly in adding the on-field motions of football players into their training, has come up with his own technique for training Julius Peppers. Arnold explains the benefits of these exercises as targeting the key muscle groups that Peppers will use while exploding through the offensive line and disrupting play in the backfield.

LONG-STRIDE DUCK WALK WITH SLED DRIVE

Arnold: The Duck Walk fatigues your explosive speed muscles—glutes, quads, hamstrings and hips—about 80 percent before you have to drive the sled. This is how it is for Julius on the field; he performs a fatiguing action, like fighting through a blocker, then he explodes into the QB or ball carrier.

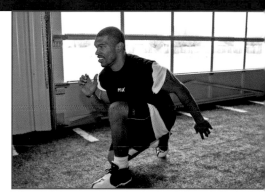

- Starting 10 yards away from sled, perform duck walk [walking crouched down with hips at knee level]

- Within one foot of sled, raise chin while maintaining low hips; pause briefly

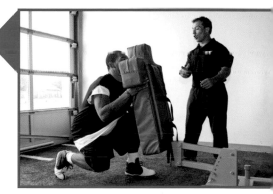

- Keeping hips low, explode into sled and drive it for three steps

COACHING POINTS

- ➤ Stay tight in hips; don't let them rise
- ➤ When exploding into sled, use hip movement you use when tackling
- ➤ Always keep chest up

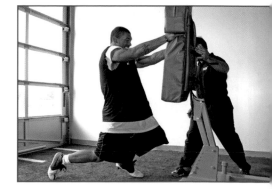

45-DEGREE LUNGE WALK WITH SLED DRIVE

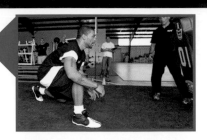

Arnold: When you reach the sled, your feet will probably be in an awkward position. Football is not played in a controlled environment, so very rarely will you be in a perfect stance. You have to be powerful and able to react and explode when your feet are not lined up perfectly underneath you.

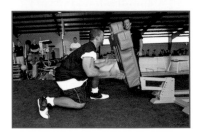

- Perform 45-degree Lunge Walk for 10 yards toward sled

- Upon reaching sled, explode into it without taking false step or adjusting feet in any way

Benefits: Improves power when legs are fatigued and in imperfect stance

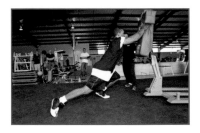

COACHING POINTS

- Keep back flat
- Do not overstride when lunging
- Do not rush drill
- Simulate same hip motion when exploding into sled as when making a tackle

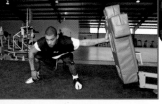

PERPENDICULAR SLED DRIVE

Arnold: The bench press movement engages your chest and shoulders, just like you would with weights; but the drill involves your whole body in a much more functional way by creating resistance similar to those you have to deal with on the field.

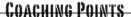

- Assume low squat position with sled arm's length to left

- Keeping hips low, pivot and explode into sled

- With hips locked out, perform explosive bench press movement with sled five times

- Repeat with sled to right

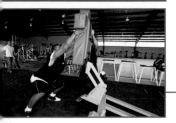

COACHING POINTS

- Keep back flat
- Do not widen stance upon contacting sled
- Bench press sled as fast as possible with control

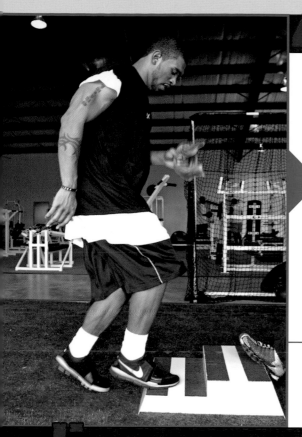

4 QUICK STEPS

Arnold: This drill creates an aerobic effect, strengthens the calves and shins, and trains fast twitch muscles—the ones used when sprinting and playing football.

- Stand in front of three- to six-inch step

- Step up with right foot, then left

- Step down with right foot, then left

- Repeat pattern as quickly as possible for specified time

- Alternate lead foot each set

COACHING POINTS

➡ Use arms to simulate running form and help move lower body

➡ Stay focused to go as quickly as possible

5 MED BALL ROTATION WITH RESISTANCE

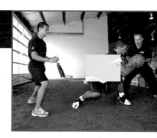

- With partner on either side, assume athletic stance holding med ball in front at shoulder level

- Without pivoting, rotate left. Keep hips low and resist as partner pushes against med ball

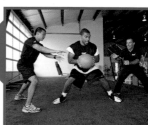

- Return to center, then rotate right, resisting as partner pushes against med ball

- Continue rotating quickly and resisting for specified reps

Advanced Modification: Perform last set with eyes closed, while partners push med ball in any direction

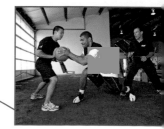

Benefits: Improves balance, core and upper-body strength

COACHING POINTS

➡ When rotating while pushing, do not lean or twist at knees

➡ Twist at waist

PARTNER STICK RESISTANCE

Arnold: This drill can bring an amazing athlete like Julius back to reality. It puts him in an incredibly vulnerable position—the same as when he is playing.

- Hold stick with shoulder-width grip and assume squat position with low center of gravity and good foot surface on ground

- Raise stick forward to shoulder level and allow partner to grasp stick outside of hands

- Without letting head or chest dip or feet come together, maintain balance and resist partner's movement as he forcefully pushes and pulls stick in all directions

Advanced Modification: Perform last set with eyes closed

Benefits: Improves balance, quickness, body awareness, power, and reaction speed while training hips and quads

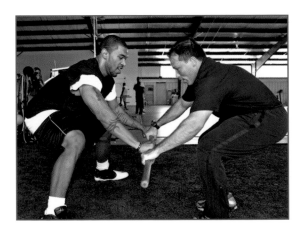 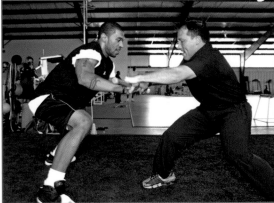

COACHING POINTS

- ➡ Keep hips low
- ➡ Move feet quickly to react to and resist partner's force
- ➡ Maintain the same body position throughout drill

CORE TRAINING

Arnold agrees that a strong core is essential to being a successful football player; but he also thinks some athletes overdo it. "The core is overemphasized these days," he says. "You see some athletes working it every day, and they get so caught up in it that before they know it, 45 minutes have gone by and they're still training their abs. So many other things could've been done in that time."

To keep Julius' core training quick and to the point, Arnold has him perform a single set of the following exercises, sometimes between working other muscle groups.

MED BALL CRUNCH WITH TOUCH

- Lie with back on ground, holding med ball with straight arms in front of chest

- As partner moves hands to various locations, crunch up and touch ball to his hands

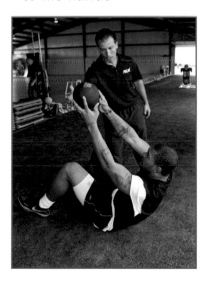
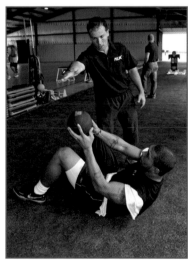
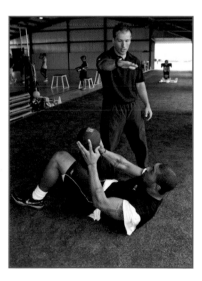

COACHING POINTS

- ➡ Keep eyes focused on partner's hands
- ➡ Do not use momentum to crunch up
- ➡ Control motion on way down
- ➡ Keep knees bent 45 degrees

2 ELBOW CRUNCH

- Lie with back and elbows on ground

- Keeping elbows on ground, perform crunch

COACHING POINTS

➤ Do not use momentum to crunch up
➤ Control motion on way down
➤ Keep knees bent 45 degrees

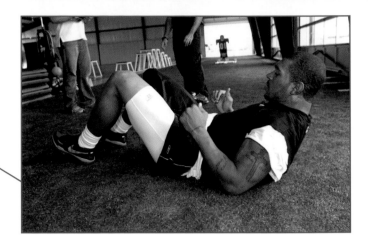

3 SIDE PLANK

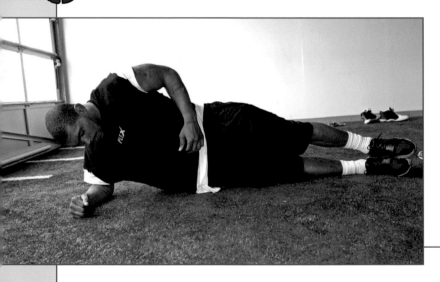

- Lie on side with elbow tucked underneath

- Raise body into side plank position so that only elbow and side of foot are touching ground

- Lower body and repeat for specified reps

COACHING POINTS

➤ Keep back flat
➤ Control body when lowering

4 MED BALL SIT-UP WITH RESISTED NEGATIVE

- Lie on back holding med ball against chest

- Perform sit-up

- Resist as partner pushes against med ball as you go back down

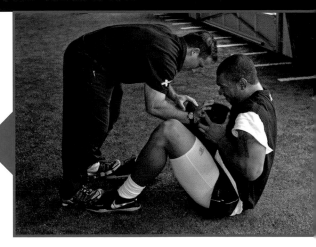

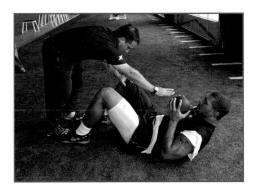

COACHING POINTS

➡ Keep knees bent 45 degrees
➡ Do not use momentum to sit up
➡ Stay controlled on way down

5 PLANK WITH HAND TOUCH

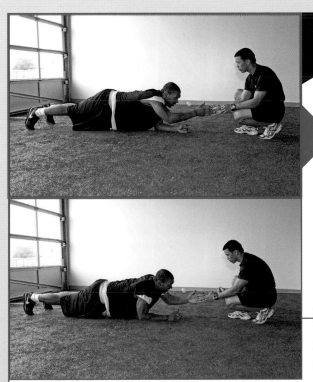

- Assume plank position on toes and elbows, with partner in front

- Keeping body in straight line, reach right hand out to touch partner's hand

- Place right elbow down; repeat with left hand

- Continue in alternating fashion for specified reps

COACHING POINTS

➡ Keep eyes focused on partner's hands ➡ Keep back flat
➡ Stay in control and slowly alternate from hand to hand

6 JACKKNIFE WITH RESISTANCE

- Lie with back on ground, knees bent 90 degrees and arms extended straight out in front of chest

- Squeeze abdominals to bring knees and arms together

- Resist as partner tries to push knees away from your arms

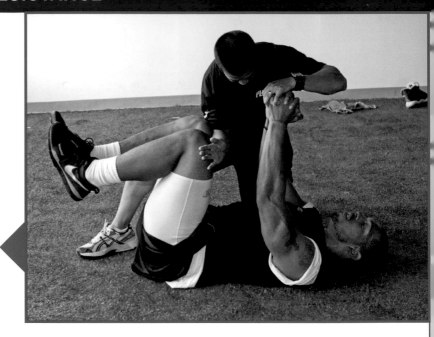

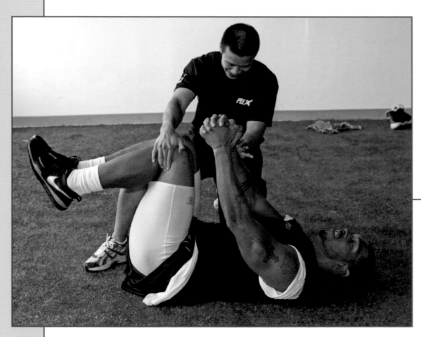

COACHING POINTS

➡ Keep knees together and bent 90 degrees

➡ Partner should push with enough strength to slowly separate hands and knees

JULIUS PEPPERS' TRAINING GUIDE

WARM UP

	SETS	REPS
Physioball Vertical Raise	3	15
Physioball Press	3	15
Band Pull-Apart	3	15
Single-Arm Dumbbell External Rotation	3	10 each arm
Single-Arm Dumbbell Raise	3	10 each arm
Opposite Hand Toe Touch	2	10 each arm and foot
Single-Arm Shoulder Balance	3	10 each arm
Basketball Wall Dribble	2	15 seconds each arm

FIELD WORK

	SETS	REPS/DISTANCE/DURATION	RECOVERY
Long-Stride Duck Walk With Sled Drive	3	10 yards	60 seconds
45-Degree Lunge Walk With Sled Drive	3	10 yards	60 seconds
Perpendicular Sled Drive	2	5 each side	60 seconds
Quick Steps	5	30 seconds	60 seconds
Med Ball Rotation With Resistance	3	10 each side	60 seconds
Partner Stick Resistance	5	10 seconds	60 seconds

CORE TRAINING

	SETS	REPS/DURATION
Med Ball Crunch With Touch	1	25
Elbow Crunch	1	25
Side Plank	1	25 each side
Med Ball Sit-Up With Resisted Negative	1	10
Plank With Hand Touch	1	20
Jackknife With Resistance	1	15 seconds

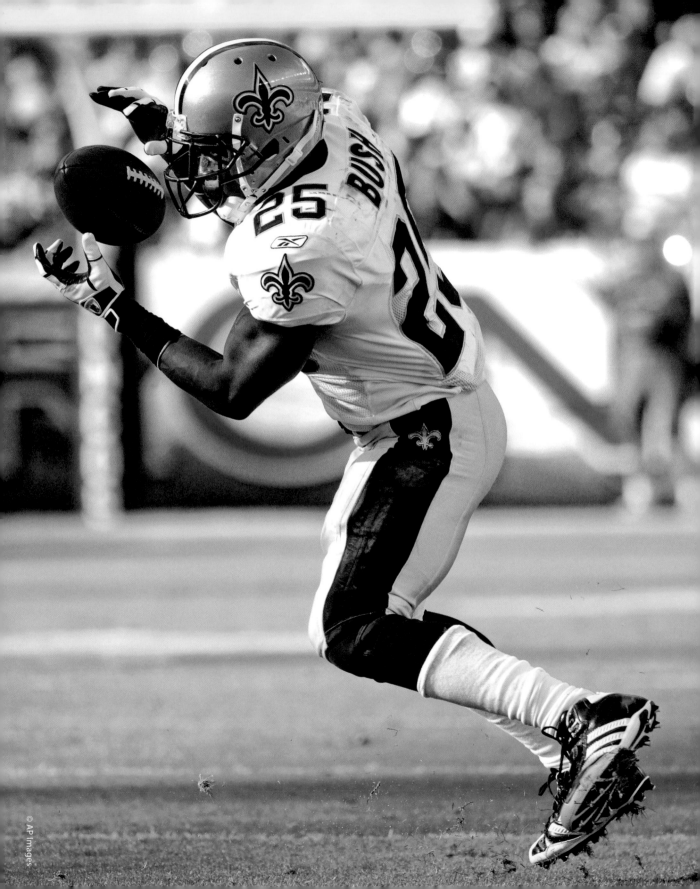

CHAPTER 5

REGGIE BUSH

EDITOR'S NOTE

We first met Reggie Bush halfway through his Heisman Trophy-winning junior year at USC. In the midst of one of the most impressive seasons in college football history—one filled with more jukes, cutbacks, and touchdowns than USC opponents care to remember—we had a chance to watch the young, explosive running back bust out an in-season lift with USC strength coach Chris Carlisle for our January 2006 cover feature. Immediately, we were impressed.

The second time we met Bush was after his athleticism and silly skills had captivated every NFL scout in the nation. At his Pro Day, we stood next to Bush as he took his stance for his 4.33-second 40-yard dash, benched 225 pounds 24 times, and exploded more than 40 inches off the turf into the beautiful Southern California sky. Observing Bush's freakish abilities so up close and personal was a truly memorable experience, as was our impeccably timed post-40 high-five—the perfect ending to an amazing day.

If you can't tell, we caught a little case of Bush infatuation, which wasn't dampened a bit after his once-invincible, chiseled body broke down following two years of NFL competition.

REGGIE BUSH WRAPS UP A SCREEN PASS DURING A GAME AGAINST THE BRONCOS IN 2008. BUSH'S COMBINATION OF SPEED AND ELUSIVENESS IS HONED DURING HIS OFF-SEASON WORKOUTS.

We knew he still worked hard every day; we knew he was still the most explosive and exciting player in the NFL; and we knew we wanted him on the cover of *STACK* Magazine—again.

So in the summer of 2008, when we learned that Bush was moving some serious iron at Elite Athletics in Westlake Village, California, we couldn't resist. It was official. Bush would be the first-ever two-time *STACK* cover athlete.

Bush greeted us for the third time with an anxious grin—smiling about the opportunity, nervous about the workout ahead of him. In a very focused and intense interview, he explained that the training he was about to do was part of achieving his overall goal for the upcoming NFL season—remaining healthy and on the field. The task would be accomplished with Travelle Gaines helping to strengthen him from head to toe, with a special focus on legs. In short, Bush wanted to be an every-down back who could move the pile and help his team win.

Although he was again sidelined by injury midway through the 2008 season, Bush's dedicated training at Elite Athletics allowed him to bounce back and return for the last few games. Over the 10 games of his injury-shortened season, he racked up 1,115 all-purpose yards and ran for nine TDs [three on kick returns].

This is Reggie Bush's cover feature from the August/September 2008 issue of *STACK* Magazine.

IRON MAN

My main motivation is to bounce back harder and stronger than ever before. That's my job; that's what I do. I play football. And when I'm done with this game, I want to be known as one of the best who ever played this position.
—Reggie Bush

When Reggie Bush left the University of Southern California in 2005, he was invincible. The most electrifying football player in the country looked like he had been carved from steel, with muscle definition seen only in cartoon superheroes. The physique and athleticism that led to a Heisman Trophy, 8.7 yards per carry, and 233 all-purpose yards per game during Bush's final season made him the NFL's next franchise-changing player.

Despite comments that he didn't have the size to compete with the NFL's monstrous power backs, the explosive burner from Southern Cal could hardly be stopped.

Simultaneously, 1,900 miles from L.A., the people of New Orleans were working hard to bounce back from the devastation of Hurricane Katrina. They needed a positive distraction, a hope of some sort. And the night before the 2006 NFL Draft, through a surprise move by the

Houston Texans, Saints fans got just that. The Texans picked defensive end Mario Williams, leaving Bush available to the Saints at No. 2.

Reggiemania erupted, as Bush t-shirts and jerseys sold at record pace. Mayor C. Ray Nagin even addressed his constituents to announce that "Saint Reggie" would be one of the major sources of hope in the region.

Accepting this role, the young back commenced his NFL career by doing what many expected. He burst onto the scene, his first TD coming on a 65-yard punt return against Tampa Bay. The arrival was not really surprising when you consider who inspired Bush's game when he was a child growing up in San Diego—two of the NFL's greatest playmakers, Deion Sanders and Barry Sanders.

Soon, Bush wasn't just a playmaker like his idols, but a game-changer for the Saints. He helped pave the Saints' way to the NFL playoffs with a key divisional win over the 49ers in which he scored four TDs [three rushing, one receiving]. Bush fueled an unlikely turnaround that brought the Saints within one game of Super Bowl XLI. New Orleans' future seemed bright.

Not so fast, Reggie. A slow start and a knee injury in 2007 put a quick stop to the resurgence. Though he attempted to battle through a slightly torn posterior cruciate ligament, the injury became too much for Bush to bear. His stats declined significantly from his promising rookie season, as he became a victim of the sophomore slump. It was the first chink in Bush's armor. "Year 1 was okay because we got to the championship game," Bush says. "This past year was the hardest thing for me to overcome in my entire career—being injured for the first time and having to miss games. I had never missed a game in my football career, whether it was Pop Warner, high school, or college. That was pretty tough for me to sit on the sidelines and watch everything happen."

Once the 2008 off-season began, Bush used as motivation how scrupulously his comeback campaign would be watched and judged. "I feel like I really need to prove myself," he says. "That's what has inspired me to work even harder and come back even stronger. This career can be short or it can be long, you never know. So you have to take every year like it's your last."

To make his mark on the '08 season, Bush tapped into his love of throwing around some serious iron in the weight room—which he says is his favorite part of training. "[During the off-season], I really focused on getting stronger," Bush says. "Coming off my injury year, I wanted

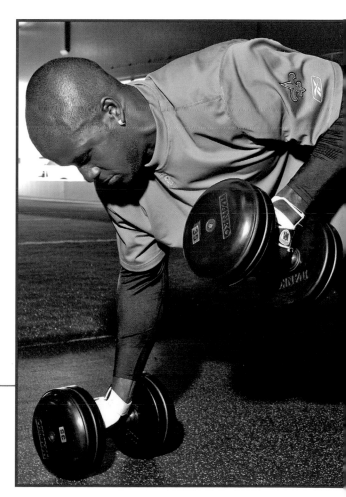

to beef up a little bit more and get stronger in that sense. It was part of the injury and me just realizing that I need to be stronger, because breaking arm tackles is very important for a running back. You get a lot of guys trying to tackle you with one arm, and I want to break those tackles."

Breaking tackles is only one of Bush's expectations. "I have team goals first, then some personal goals," he says. "One of those team goals is to always win at home. [After that], win our divisional games, get to the playoffs, [then] the Super Bowl.

"For personal goals, I look to get to the Pro Bowl and rush for somewhere between 1,500 and 2,000 yards. Just to be one of the top backs in the league and be very productive game in and game out."

The desire to beef up and achieve those lofty goals led Bush back to Southern California and the Elite Athletics training facility, owned by teammate Billy Miller. For the crucial six weeks before training camp, Bush worked with Elite's director of pro athlete development, Travelle Gaines, who was impressed with Bush from the get-go. "I mean, Reggie is one of the best athletes in the world," Gaines says. "He is such a goal-oriented person that sets very high standards for himself. After a two-hour workout, he'll stay for an additional hour of work on his own. I have never met a person who loved lifting weights or who enjoys being in the gym more than Reggie."

Each day Bush showed up at Elite Athletics, he faced an intense, total-body training session. And nothing made him happier, because he was one step closer to becoming the strong, tackle-breaking back he set out to be. "From the time Reggie started earlier this summer until [the final few weeks of training], he's made a dramatic improvement," Gaines recalls. "He would come in every day, ready for the challenge to get better. And you would see a different person each day. You could see him transforming into the person and athlete he wanted to be. I figured out that any time you take God-given ability and add hard work, you get a player like Reggie Bush— and very rarely does that come around."

Don't be surprised if you see No. 25 dash between the tackles on an inside run, explode through a tackler, then move the pile after contact. That's his job; that's what he does.

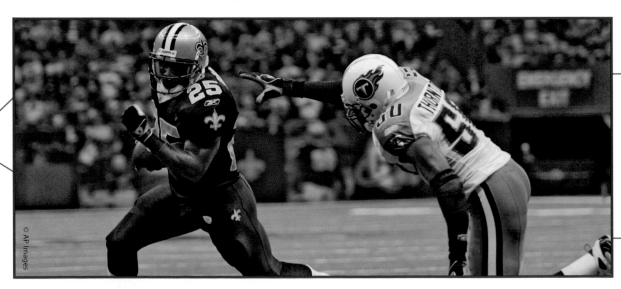

© AP Images

PREHAB RESISTANCE SERIES

Before Bush starts his intense strength training, Gaines works to get his upper-body muscles firing as quickly as possible. These prehab exercises prepare Bush's chest, upper back, shoulders, and traps, so he can tackle the explosive movements that follow.

Gaines says, "We focus on this region because you see so many shoulder injuries in football. Players need to be strong there because they get hit there so often."

PRESS

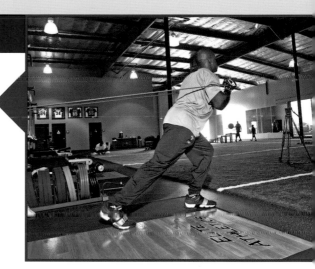

- With light band resistance attached to stable object behind you, step forward into staggered position

- Hold handles at chest so band has tension

- Continuously punch arms forward and back as fast as possible for specified duration

COACHING POINTS

➤ Make sure back leg is straight and front leg is slightly bent, similar to wide receiver's stance

➤ Focus on punching straight out, coming straight back and pressing to full extension

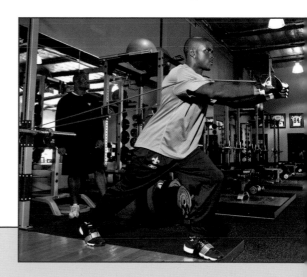

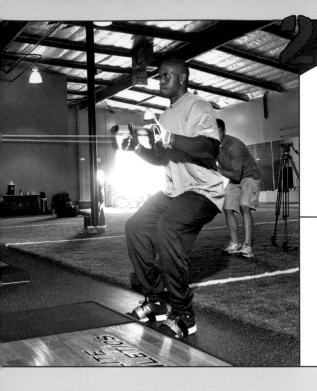

ROW

- With light band resistance attached to stable object in front, step back into even stance, creating tension in band

- Continuously drive elbows back and forth for specified duration

COACHING POINTS

- Focus on body position, pushing butt back [into sitting position] and keeping chest up
- Squeeze shoulder blades together when rowing
- Do not allow form to deteriorate after initial 20 seconds

REAR SHOULDER

- With light band resistance in front, step back into even stance

- Hold handles so arms are straight in front and band has tension

- Keeping arms straight, bring handles back and overhead into V position; return arms to start position

- Repeat movement as fast as possible for specified duration

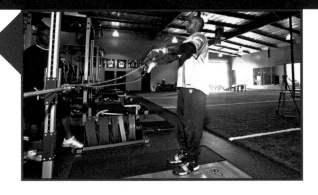

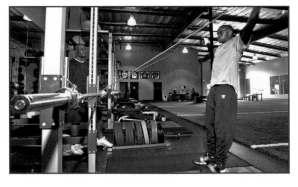

COACHING POINTS

- Stand straight up
- Bring arms straight out to 45 degrees

RESISTANCE TRAINING

Finally, Gaines works Bush out with some resistance training—not only to strengthen his body, but also as a speed endurance workout, which is necessary for Bush to gain strength without losing speed. Reggie performs exercise **1A** for strength, then supersets it with **1B** to work endurance. Exercise **2** hits on speed, strength, and endurance.

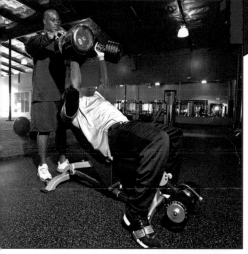

1A ALTERNATE DUMBBELL INCLINE PRESS

Gaines: We make sure Reggie keeps his arms turned in a punching motion, because there's never a time in football when your arms should be out wide. You're probably holding if they are out there. You have to be explosive and tight from the armpit and be able to punch straight up. This is a great stabilization exercise for upper-body muscles.

- Lie with back on incline bench, holding dumbbells with palms facing each other at upper chest

- Extend both arms toward ceiling, keeping palms facing in

- Keeping left arm locked out, lower right dumbbell to chest, then punch it toward ceiling

- Keeping right arm locked out, lower left dumbbell to chest, then punch it toward ceiling

- Repeat sequence for specified reps

COACHING POINTS

➤ Keep arms facing in throughout exercise
➤ Keep opposite arm locked out in tight position, not wide

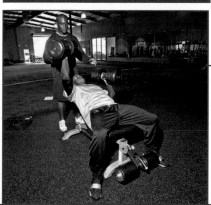

PUSH-UP TO ROW

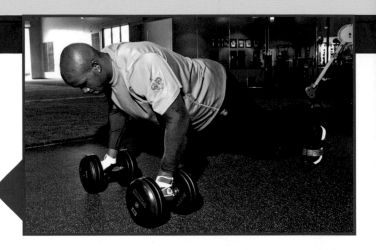

Gaines: This helps tremendously with core stability, because it gets Reggie into an awkward position where he has to balance himself. On the football field, you are never in a standard position, where your weight is equally balanced.

- Assume push-up position with light dumbbells in hands

- Perform push-up, then row with right arm

- Perform push-up then row with left arm

- Repeat sequence for specified reps

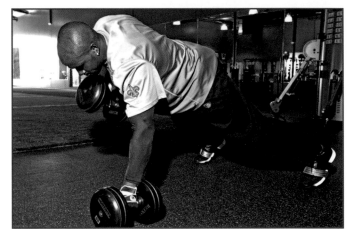

COACHING POINTS

- Perform immediately after set of Alternating Dumbbell Incline Press
- Get into a good push-up position with legs spread about shoulder width
- Drive your arm up as high as possible and close to breastplate when rowing
- Focus on keeping body in stable position

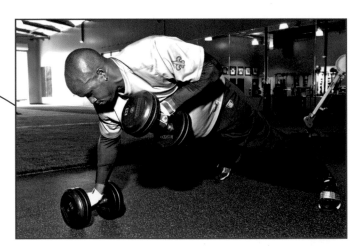

CONE TOUCH WITH RESISTANCE

Gaines: We do this with Reggie [to] get him sprinting forward and really force him to dig because of the resistance. As the resistance increases, he has to pump his arms and legs more violently and concentrate on his form. His body is being propelled backwards, so he is forced to squeeze his ab muscles to control his body. It improves body control and [helps him learn to] deal with resistance, very similar to dragging a defender. This will definitely help him shed tacklers.

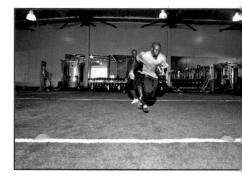

- Place two cones five yards apart, five yards in front of you

- Assume athletic stance with partner providing band resistance from behind

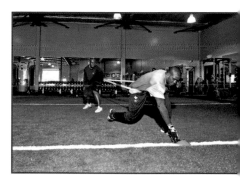

- Holding football in left hand, explode forward at angle toward left cone, bend at waist, touch cone with right hand

- Backpedal with control to start position

- Transfer ball to right hand, then explode forward at angle to right cone

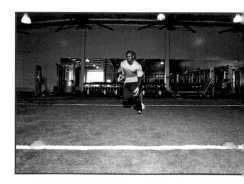

- Touch cone with left hand, then backpedal with control to start position

- Repeat in continuous fashion for specified duration

COACHING POINTS

➤ Keep resistance moderate to avoid poor form and straining

➤ Pump arms and legs to explode against resistance

➤ Bend at waist to touch cone

➤ Maintain body control on way back

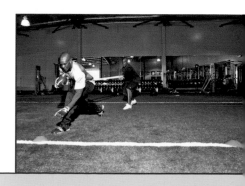

CORE CIRCUIT

Bush completes the following four core exercises as a superset, repeating the circuit four times. Not only does this strengthen his core, it is a great warm-up, according to Gaines.

OVERHEAD MED BALL THROWS

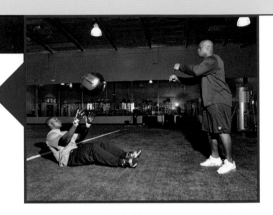

- Assume sit-up position, facing partner with med ball

- As partner throws ball, catch it and lower into sit-up

- Throw ball back to partner halfway up sit-up motion

- Repeat for specified reps

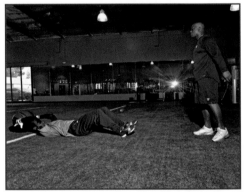

Benefits: Overall strengthening of the full frontal abdominal area, resulting in a more athletic running back

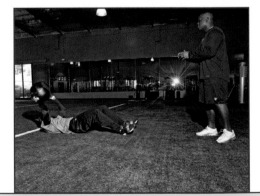

COACHING POINTS

- ➡ Dig heels into ground
- ➡ Keep ball as high above head as possible
- ➡ Throw ball back when halfway up in a continuous motion

ELITE AB THROWS

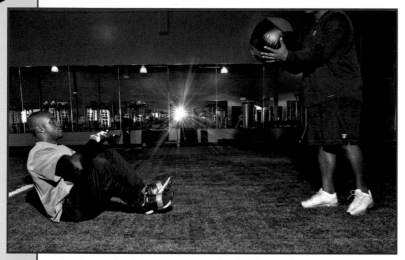

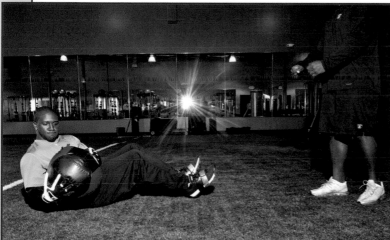

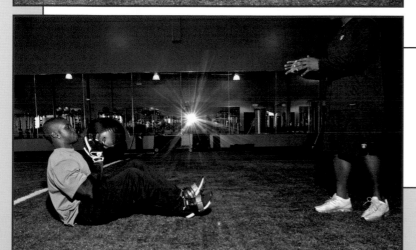

Gaines: I tell Reggie to follow the ball with his eyes to get more of a twist and work more of the oblique muscles. [I] want [him] to get full extension when he throws the ball back from his chest to help warm up his upper-body muscles. It is important for a running back like Reggie to have strong obliques, because he is always twisting and turning and trying to break tackles.

- Assume sit-up position, facing partner with med ball

- Catch ball from partner's throw; rotate right, then left

- Throw ball back to partner in explosive motion

- Repeat for specified reps

COACHING POINTS

➤ Focus eyes on ball to help rotate body

➤ Use obliques to rotate left and right

➤ Make sure ball touches ground when rotating

3 SIDE MED BALL TOSS

Gaines: Given [how] Reggie bends and navigates his body through the field, he needs to be strong in the obliques.

- Assume sit-up position with partner to left

- As partner throws ball from side, catch it and rotate right

- Touch ball to ground; immediately and explosively throw ball back to partner rotating left

- Repeat for specified reps; perform set on opposite side

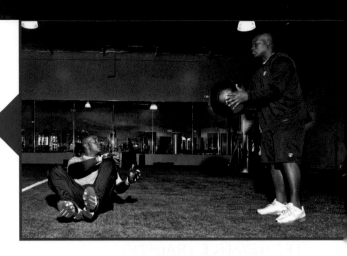

COACHING POINTS

➤ Follow ball with eyes
➤ Catch ball in front of body
➤ Throw ball back as soon at it touches ground, in one explosive movement

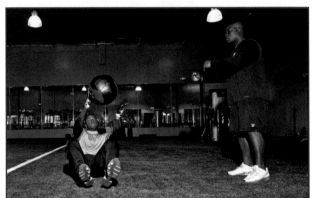

4 PHYSIOBALL JACKKNIFE

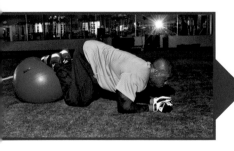

Gaines: This hits the bottom half of the abs and also helps Reggie's overall core stability and strength, which gives him a better foundation. You need a phenomenal core to be a great athlete in general. I have Reggie focus on making sure he keeps his body in a stable position while driving his knees as high as possible.

- Assume push-up position with feet on top of physioball

- Keeping body stable, roll physioball toward hands by driving knees as high as possible and digging toes into ball

- Return legs to full extension; repeat in controlled fashion for specified reps

COACHING POINTS

➤ Dig toes into top of physioball ➤ Drive knees up as high as possible
➤ Get full extension with legs when rolling ball out ➤ Focus on stabilizing the body with arms

REGGIE BUSH'S TRAINING GUIDE

PREHAB RESISTANCE SERIES

	SETS	REPS
Press	2	30 seconds
Row	2	30 seconds
Rear Shoulder	2	30 seconds

RESISTANCE TRAINING

	SETS	REST
Alternate Dumbbell Incline Press*	4	10 each arm
Push-Up to Row*	4	8 each arm
Cone Touch With Resistance	4	30 seconds

*Superset

CORE CIRCUIT

Beginners: Use 6-pound med ball
High schoolers: Use 10- to 12-pound med ball
College and professional athletes: Use 12- to 14-pound med ball

	SETS	REPS
Overhead Med Ball Throws	4	15
Elite Ab Throws	4	15
Side Med Ball Toss	4	10 each side
Physioball Jackknife	4	15

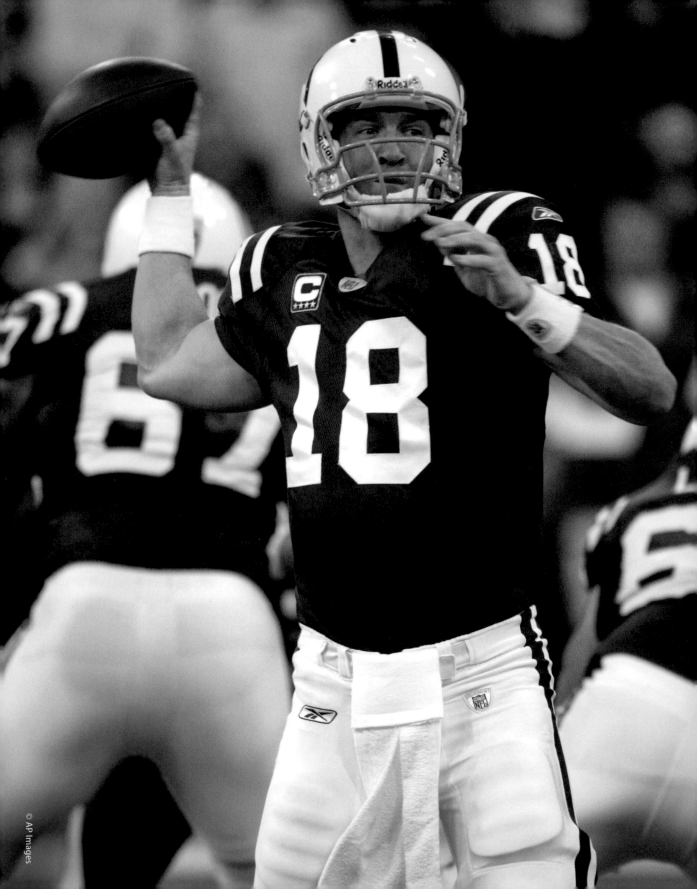

CHAPTER 6

PEYTON MANNING

EDITOR'S NOTE

During the summer of 2007, Peyton Manning was coming off a Super Bowl championship and MVP Award. When we sat down to decide which football player to kick off our year with, the discussion did not last very long. Manning was on top of the football world in every way.

In the midst of his post-championship hoopla, Manning found the time, together with his former University of Tennessee teammate Will Bartholomew, to open a new D1 Sports Training facility in Chattanooga, Tennessee. Their goal was to provide the brutal-but-effective training they had discovered at the University of Tennessee to high school, college, and other professional athletes. But Manning did more than lend his name to the facility; he turned his body over to Bartholomew and the D1 staff.

On a muggy summer afternoon, we showed up at D1 expecting to see a slightly heavier, relaxed, and tanned Peyton Manning, fresh off some banquet or parade, tossing the football around for a little off-season "workout." Instead, Manning arrived on time, with purpose, and wearing his usual intense scowl, and proceeded to bust his ass for 60 straight minutes. The rest between sets

PEYTON MANNING, SHOWN HERE DURING A GAME IN 2008, HAS USED AN INTENSIVE TRAINING PROGRAM TO BUILD ENDURANCE FOR THE LONG NFL SEASON.

and exercises was so brief that Manning barely had time to bend down, pick up a towel, and wipe his sweat-drenched face. He also didn't smile at all, but that may have been more by choice.

The focus of Manning's training caught us off guard as well. He performed a variety of explosive medicine ball exercises and agility drills—then pumped iron. It's probably not what you'd expect from a champion star quarterback. At one point, he was busting out reps on the bench with 90-pound dumbbells. We silently apologized for previously mocking how quarterbacks trained.

During our post-workout conversation, Manning talked mostly about his family support, All-Pro upbringing, and hunger for another Super Bowl title. Although the Colts have not yet accomplished that, Manning has continued to distinguish himself as the game's best signal caller. Most recently, he took home the NFL's 2008 MVP Award; but judging from our encounter with the 6'5", 230-pound perfectionist, we have a feeling he's not satisfied with that alone.

The following is Peyton Manning's cover feature from the August/September 2007 issue of *STACK* Magazine.

BACK FOR MORE

They say you can judge a man's character by the way he handles defeat. But you can learn just as much about a man and his heart by looking at how he responds to success and the accomplishment of his ultimate goals.

We've all witnessed a Super Bowl champion fall from grace after earning his title, never to reach that pinnacle again. Blame it on complacency, or point to the dismantling of his talented supporting cast. Either way, the brand of effort and hard work that produced the hero's championship run somehow got lost during his visits to the White House, TV appearances, and victory parades.

Football analysts around the country are waiting to see if Super Bowl XLI MVP Peyton Manning succumbs to one of these post-championship tailspins. We didn't want to sit and wonder. So we asked Manning straight up if hard work has taken a back seat to a long, gratifying victory lap. Firmly, he reminded us how he refused to rest on the laurels of his record-breaking 49 TD passes in '04, or dwell on disappointment after the Patriots and Steelers ended his seasons prematurely in consecutive AFC Championship games. So why would he let himself lose focus now that he's on top?

"I got some advice from Derrick Brooks, the great linebacker from Tampa Bay who finally won a Super Bowl in his 10th or 11th year," Manning says. "He told me to enjoy this experience and not hurry to put it all behind me, but still work as hard this off-season as I did last year. I've done that and then some."

Taking Brooks' advice, Manning has relished the glory that comes with a Super Bowl victory, but he cherishes the less-publicized rewards the most. "This has been a very enjoyable off-season for me, but the best times have been with my teammates—the guys who helped us win Super Bowl XLI," Manning says. "Whether I'm out to dinner with Dallas Clark and Jeff Saturday, or lifting weights with Marvin Harrison and Reggie Wayne, there's always that moment, between sets of bench press or just sitting in the restaurant, when we make eye contact and know what we accomplished last year and how hard we worked to accomplish it."

Hungry for more, Manning and his teammates recognize the level of effort they need to match last year's success. "We've been working a long time for this; it was nice to finally accomplish our ultimate goal," he says. "And once we did, it made us want to go out and do it again. We know what it takes."

Don't expect to catch a glimpse of Manning's Super Bowl ring while he's working for the next title; it's not his style. "I won't wear [my ring] out much. I'll probably lock it up somewhere safe," he says. "When you win the Super Bowl, you know it in your heart and mind. You don't have to wear something that tells everyone you did it."

All-Pro Upbringing

In previous seasons, Manning used his uncanny focus and hard work to battle through the most gut-wrenching disappointments. These same qualities—nurtured during his youth in New Orleans—are now guiding him through his post-championship existence.

Growing up under the tutelage of storied NFL quarterback Archie Manning taught Peyton more than just passing skills. "My father always told me, 'If you want to accomplish anything in this lifetime, you've got to have a strong work ethic and never lose sight of your goal,'" Manning says. "That applied to school, sports, or trying to make myself a better athlete. I always had to take care of my schoolwork and other responsibilities before sports."

Although born weighing 12 pounds, and into a football family, Manning was not immediately handed a pigskin and sent off to practice. "I grew up in a football environment, but I was fortunate that my dad never pushed me into sports," he says. "He encouraged me and my brothers to play sports because it teaches you to overcome challenges, work with teammates, and take coaching, but it was never a pressure situation. Our philosophy was that if

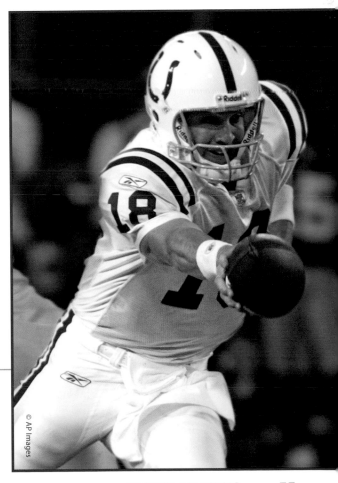

© AP Images

we wanted help, we had to go to him and ask for it. That was a healthy way to do it."

By the age of three, Manning apparently knew his athletic destiny, as he was waddling around the Manning family's backyard and heaving passes to his brother. About a decade later, when he reached the age of competitive play, Manning sought the help he knew was available. "When I was in junior high, I wanted to be the quarterback on my middle school's seventh grade team," Manning recalls. "I had this great ex-quarterback in my house, so I milked him for as much knowledge as I could. I asked for help, and he started coming to watch my brother and me work out on the field."

This NFL-caliber coaching, combined with his QB pedigree, had coaches drooling by the time Manning entered high school. Heading into his sophomore season at Isidore Newman, he was handed the reins as starting quarterback, although his older brother Cooper was slated to call plays for the Greenies that year—his senior season. Making a potentially bad situation positive, Cooper moved to wide receiver and became Manning's favorite target. Manning recalls the experience with fondness: "When Cooper became my wide receiver, we'd go out and work on the field. I really miss those times in high school and all the great memories."

Filling Out

While Manning possessed big-time skills as a passer, his body was not exactly up to speed.

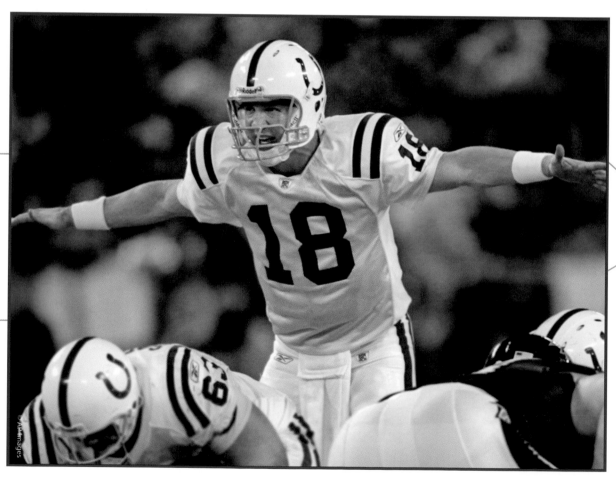

"I grew five inches in one year in high school," he says. "I was tall, skinny, and slow. I don't think I could run out of sight in a week." So Manning began intense weightlifting sessions in addition to watching hours of film. From that point on, his dedication to his body never dwindled, and he remained well ahead of the competition and other quarterbacks.

At the University of Tennessee, it didn't take Manning long to solidify his reputation as a workout freak with his teammates. Eventually, he became the Volunteers' best QB of all time, literally rewriting the record books. During his senior campaign, Manning set UT's single-season mark for completions (287), passing yards (3,819), and touchdowns (36)—the triple crown of passing.

After nine seasons with the Colts, Manning has finally shut up his critics, who had been clamoring that he couldn't win the big one. Now, besides being the best quarterback in football and the leader of the best team in the league, Manning still possesses the work ethic that turned his awkward body into a 6'5", 230-pound rocket-armed passing machine.

D1 Training

Manning first met Will Bartholomew, president and CEO of D1 Sports Training, at the University of Tennessee. "I was trying to recruit Will to play football for Tennessee," Manning says. "It wasn't a hard sell since his daddy and grandpa went there. I think he's been a Volunteer since birth."

While Manning gained fame as a QB, Bartholomew blazed a stellar career as a fullback, eventually captaining the squad in 2001. As the two pushed through excruciating weight room sessions together, they gained a mutual respect for each other and realized a common interest.

After an injury-shortened stint with the Denver Broncos, Bartholomew set his sights on helping other athletes reach their goals, giving birth to the D1 Training philosophy. Shortly thereafter, he brought Manning on board. "Will approached me about three years ago about his philosophy and ideas about helping athletes get better," Manning says. "Will and I were always doing everything we could to make ourselves better athletes on the field and in the weight room, so it seemed like a natural fit." By 2005, Manning was a member of the D1 family as the co-owner of one of the facilities; he now owns three.

With strong faith in D1's philosophy, Manning turns his body over to Bartholomew and his staff every off-season. "Will named it D1—not because he can guarantee that you will become a D-I athlete—but because he will train you like one," Manning says. "They hold you accountable for yourself, and you're truly part of a team here. I wish I had something like this when I was 14 years old. Back then, I saw some crazy exercises on TV and would go do them in my backyard. I had no idea what I was doing. We would lift weights, and then have to drive across town for a field to run on. Here, they have weights and the field."

D1 has helped countless athletes reach their ultimate goals through improved athleticism; and their most notable client is no exception. "Manning has really evolved over time with his movement in the pocket," Bartholomew recalls. "If you watch him on Sundays, you can see how powerfully and quickly he gets back on his drops. No one can drop back and get rid of the ball quicker than him."

Manning agrees: "I am a much quicker, faster, and stronger athlete as a result of my work here."

"We don't guarantee anything, but most of our athletes can expect to drop their 40 time by at least two tenths of second throughout our 12-week cycle," Bartholomew says. "That's on top of an average weight increase of 25 to 30 pounds on strength staples, like the bench press."

Although he's at the top of the football world, Manning is still looking for ways to improve his game at D1. "I'm going into my 10th year in the NFL, and I've always tried to work harder each year to be a better athlete, quarterback, and player than I was the year before," he says. "As I get older, I have to work a little harder to get better, and that's what I'm doing here."

On this particular day at the Chattanooga-based facility, the D1 staff keeps Manning moving from the second he steps out of the locker room. "This is a different kind of training than what most people are used to," he says. "When I'm working out at D1, we have the same training intensity and tempo I had back at Tennessee."

The workout begins with a quick core and flexibility session that has Manning drenched in sweat almost immediately. Then, after he's loose and solid through the core, the real improvement takes place in the form of rapid-fire agility drills and old-school iron pumping—the meat of the training. As Manning moves from station to station, it's clear that he has no plans to stop at one title.

Here is his plan to add to his trophy case.

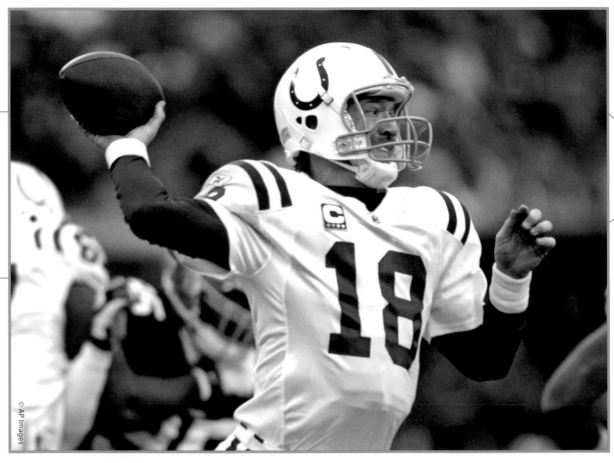

© AP Images

CORE

Bartholomew: Peyton needs to work his core, because he takes a lot of hits. A strong core helps him absorb them. It also allows him to throw at the high velocity that he does. The most important thing about training your core is to use proper form and make sure you're not rushing through the exercises. If you get going too fast, you aren't going to strengthen those muscles, and you can cause injury.

1 MED BALL TOE TOUCHES

- Lie on back with legs straight up, toes pointing toward ceiling

- Hold med ball in front of chest and crunch up until ball touches toes

- Lower with control and repeat for specified reps

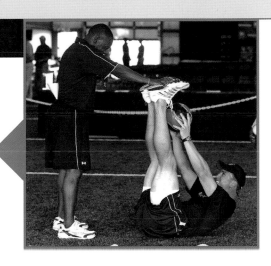

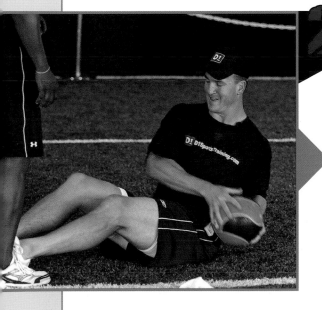

2 RUSSIAN TWIST

- Sit on ground with knees bent and just off floor

- Holding med ball in front of chest, rotate to left until ball touches floor outside left hip

- Rotate to right until ball touches floor outside right hip

- Repeat in controlled manner for specified reps

3 SEATED OVERHEAD MED BALL THROWS

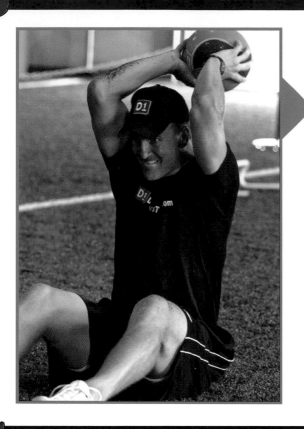

- Sit on ground with knees bent and heels just off floor

- Without changing position of upper body, receive ball from partner overhead and throw it back

- Repeat for specified reps

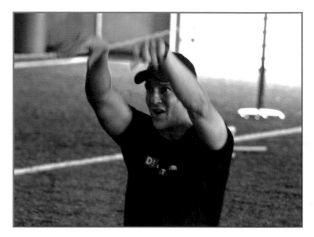

4 PARTNER MED BALL ROTATION THROWS

- Assume athletic stance with partner five yards in front

- Receive ball from partner, rotate right and throw ball back to partner with maximum force

- Perform next rep on left side

- Continue in alternating fashion for specified reps

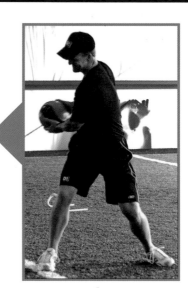
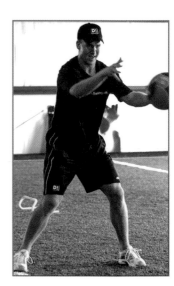

- Assume athletic stance with partner to your left

- Receive ball from partner, rotate right, then throw ball back to partner by pushing with right hand

- Repeat for specified reps; perform set on opposite side

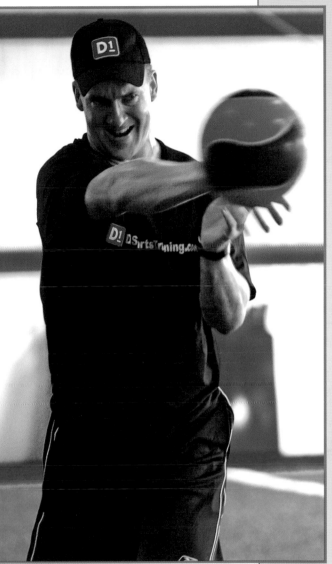

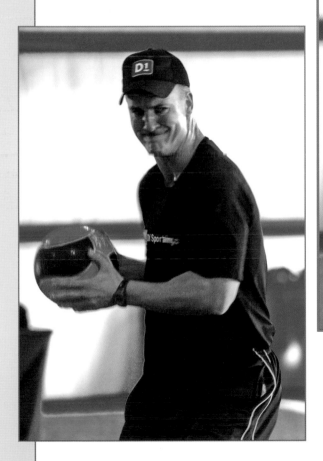

FLEXIBILITY

Bartholomew: We like to get a nice, quick stretch with Peyton as part of his warm-up. We are making sure to open up his hips and really stretch his hamstrings, so that when he goes on to his agility work, he's ready to go and doesn't pull anything. Since this is prior to working out, we're not going to hold the stretches very long. We hold each for about 15 seconds, instead of 30 to 45 like we would at the end of a workout.

STRETCHES

1. Partner Hamstring/Low Back Stretch With Shakeout

2. Partner Hamstring Stretch

3. Partner Straddle Stretch

4. Partner Quad Stretch

5. Partner Butterfly Stretch

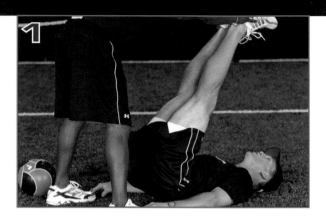

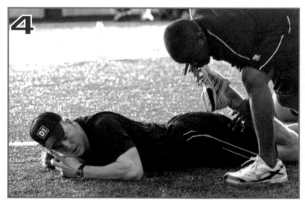

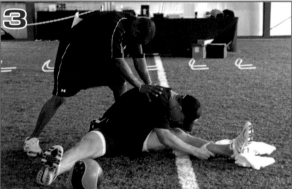

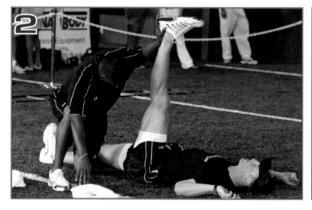

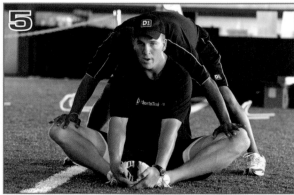

AGILITY

MINI HURDLE SHUFFLE

Bartholomew: This is great for Peyton, because he wants to keep his feet spread in the pocket at all times, so that he can throw the ball as soon as he sees an open receiver.

- Set up eight mini hurdles in row, each one foot apart

- With back to row of hurdles, assume pocket stance with ball high, knees slightly bent, and eyes downfield (over left shoulder for right-handed QBs)

- Without allowing feet to come together, shuffle backward with small steps, in and out of hurdles

- Upon reaching end of row, shuffle forward in and out of hurdles

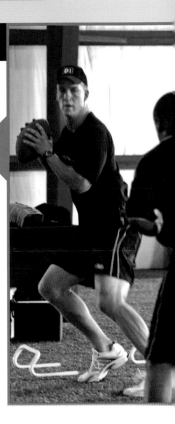

Advanced: Have partner stand downfield providing visual cues. Change direction as he points to his left or right

COACHING POINTS

➡ Do not allow feet to come together

➡ Keep hips low

REACTIVE TENNIS BALL SHUFFLE

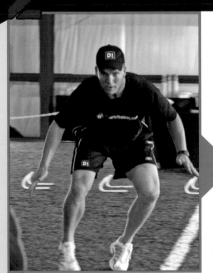

Bartholomew: This improves agility and strengthens the hips and core, helping Peyton explode out of any type of situation and react to anything that might happen on the field.

- Assume athletic stance facing partner five yards away

- As partner rolls tennis ball left and right, continuously shuffle in each direction

- Lower hips, retrieve ball and throw it back to partner

COACHING POINTS

➡ Keep hips low ➡ Don't allow feet to come together

3 PASS DROP WITH BUNGEE RESISTANCE

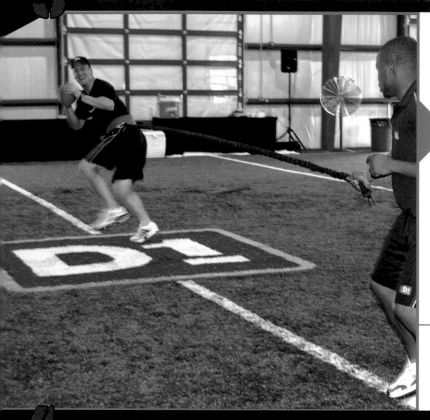

- Perform pass drop with partner providing resistance from front with bungee

- Upon setting up, step up in pocket, keeping eyes downfield

- Shuffle from side to side as though you were avoiding pass rush

- Tuck ball and sprint toward partner

COACHING POINTS

➡ Get full stride distance, and push off with front leg on each step to improve speed and power in a five-step drop

4 PASS DROP WITH OVERSPEED

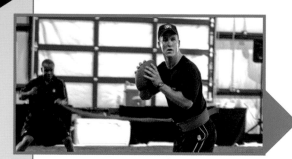

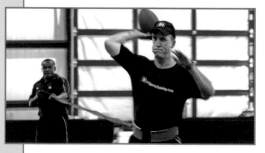

Bartholomew: The overspeed allows Peyton to get back into his drop faster than he could normally. This helps him communicate speed and quickness to his muscles and mind. Peyton can get back faster than anyone, because he can plant on the back foot and get the throw out.

- Perform pass drop with partner providing assistance from behind with bungee

- Upon setting up, step up in pocket against resistance

- Shuffle from side to side as though you were avoiding pass rush

- Simulate pass downfield

STRENGTH

DUMBBELL BENCH

Bartholomew: This is a great exercise for Peyton and any QB, because it strengthens their arms independently. Peyton is dominant with his right arm, since he is always throwing with it, so this makes sure that he's strengthening his left arm as well.

- Lie with back on bench holding dumbbells near shoulders

- Keeping elbows tight to ribs, drive dumbbells to ceiling until arms are straight

- Lower dumbbells to start position with control; repeat for specified reps

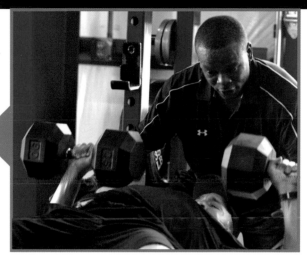

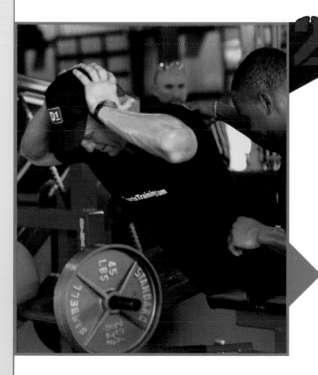

BACK HYPERS

Bartholomew: This strengthens Peyton's back, glutes and core so that he will have enough strength to withstand any kind of blow or awkward movement.

- Assume position on back hyper machine with legs locked into place and body bent 90 degrees

- Raise upper body until chest is parallel to ground

- Lower with control; repeat for specified reps

3 TRICEP PUSHDOWN DROPSET

Bartholomew: This is great for strength and strength endurance in the triceps.

- Perform 10 tricep pushdowns keeping elbows tight to ribs

- Decrease weight 10 to 15 pounds and immediately perform 10 more reps

- Decrease weight again about 10 to 15 pounds and immediately perform 10 more reps

COACHING POINTS

➡ Make sure to keep proper form all the way through dropset

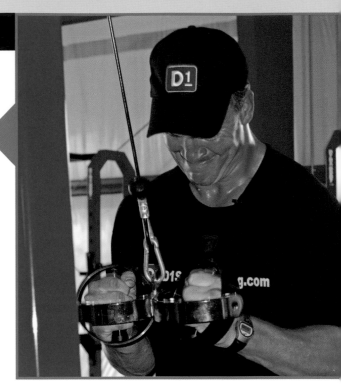

4 HAMSTRING CURL WITH SINGLE-LEG NEGATIVE

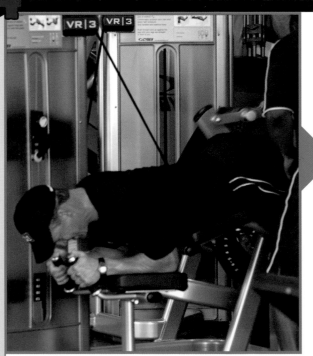

Bartholomew: This works the hamstrings explosively on the way up and then works the strength aspect as you lower the weight slowly with one leg. This helps Peyton fire his hamstrings explosively with speed, power and strength when he's running.

- Lie on hamstring curl machine with legs locked under pad

- Explosively contract hamstrings by curling both heels to butt

- Lower weight with control using only right leg until leg is straight

- Repeat for specified reps; perform set with left leg

PEYTON MANNING'S TRAINING GUIDE

CORE

Perform one core exercise, immediately followed by a flexibility exercise.
Continue supersetting until all exercises are performed.

	SETS	REPS
Med Ball Toe Touches	1	15
Russian Twist	1	10 each side
Seated Overhead Med Ball Throws	1	15
Partner Med Ball Rotation Throws	1	8 each side
Lateral Partner Med Ball Rotation Throws	1	8 each side

FLEXIBILITY

Have partner bring each stretch to a point of slight tension, then hold.
Perform directional stretches to both sides.

	SETS	DURATION
Partner Hamstring/Low Back Stretch With Shakeout	1	15 seconds
Partner Hamstring Stretch	1	15 seconds each leg
Partner Straddle Stretch (Right, Left, Center)	1	15 seconds each direction
Partner Quad Stretch	1	15 seconds each leg
Partner Butterfly Stretch	1	15 seconds

AGILITY

	SETS	REPS
Mini Hurdle Shuffle	4	5 changes of direction
Reactive Tennis Ball Shuffle	3	15 seconds
Pass Drop With Bungee Resistance	1	4
Pass Drop With Overspeed	1	4

STRENGTH

	SETS	REPS
Dumbbell Bench*	4	6
Back Hypers*	3	8-10
Tricep Pushdown Dropset*	2	10 + 10 + 10
Hamstring Curl With Single-Leg Negative*	2 each leg	5 each leg

*Superset

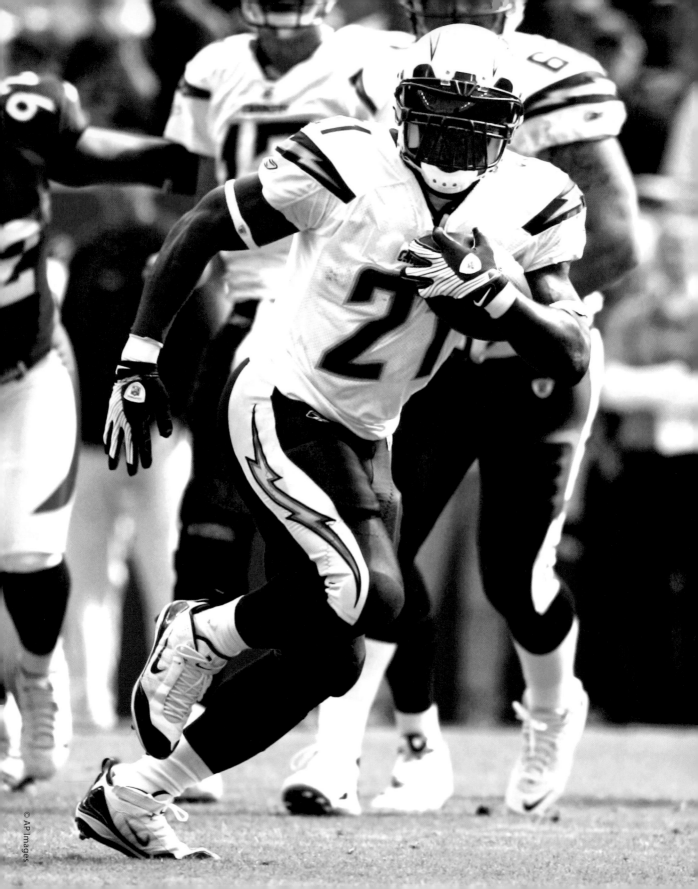

CHAPTER 7

LaDAINIAN
TOMLINSON

EDITOR'S NOTE

Back in the summer of 2005, when we began our search for the best strength and conditioning coaches—who trained the best athletes in the world—Todd Durkin, owner of Fitness Quest 10 in San Diego, California, had one of the best resumes out there. Having trained the likes of NFL studs LaDainian Tomlinson, Drew Brees, Carson Palmer, Kellen Winslow Jr., Quentin Jammer, and Will Demps, to name a few, Durkin had cemented his status among the industry's elite. Further burnishing his credentials, Durkin is a two-time Personal Trainer of the Year recipient.

When we spoke with Durkin, he graciously opened his training vault to provide us with excerpts from the functional sports performance training and speed, agility, and quickness work of one of his prized clients: Tomlinson, the five-time Pro Bowl running back. Including this information in our top 10 favorite football workouts was a no-brainer.

At the time, Tomlinson was entering his fifth year in the league with the San Diego Chargers, coming off his fourth consecutive 1,000-yard season, and extending his all-time record for most consecutive games scoring a rushing touchdown to 18. Tomlinson had become the quintessential

LADAINIAN TOMLINSON'S WORK ETHIC AND TRAINING HAVE HELPED HIM SURVIVE IN THE NFL. THE 2006 NFL MVP IS SHOWN HERE CARRYING THE BALL IN 2008.

stud back in 2003, when he was the first player in NFL history to haul in 100 receptions and rush for 1,000 yards in the same season. During his 2006 campaign, he set three NFL records with 31 total TDs, 28 rushing TDs, and most points in a season (186). He topped it off by claiming the NFL's Most Valuable Player Award.

Tomlinson's training regimen has enabled him to play at a high level and avoid serious injury. It's not often that we, as fans, get to witness a legendary running back for more than a few years. But thanks to his work ethic and dedication to training, Tomlinson has made sure he's an exception.

The following pages present an updated version of Tomlinson's cover feature article, originally published in the September 2005 issue of *STACK* Magazine. Included in the article are Durkin's training goals for Tomlinson, plus his comments on the training itself and the extraordinary athlete who performs it.

DEFYING THE ODDS

As the average lifespan of an NFL running back has dwindled down to a measly four years, LaDainian Tomlinson has defied the odds, making himself into one of the most electrifying backs in the league during his eight seasons. Before LT was selected by the San Diego Chargers—fifth overall in the 2001 NFL Draft—no back had ever delivered such a complete package of Pro Bowl-quality running, catching, blocking, and durability.

Defying odds is something LT has had to do since his childhood in Rosebud, Texas. When he was seven years old, his parents divorced and his dad left the family. Forced to raise LT and his two younger siblings on her own, his mom relied on LT to do the right things—such as instilling faith, integrity, and hard work in his brother and sister. When other kids his age were partying, LT became a responsible man, in part by combining his mom's values with his love of football.

Although he ultimately landed a football scholarship, it wasn't at a BCS school, which added fuel to LT's fire to prove he belonged.

Playing his college ball at Texas Christian University, the elusive Horned Frog put up numbers that confounded conventional expectations. In his junior year, he ran for 1,850 yards and 18 touchdowns. And in his senior campaign, he bested that output with 2,158 yards and 22 touchdowns, earning the Doak Walker Award as the nation's top running back.

No one doubted that LT had the speed and quickness to be an NFL running back, but scouts wondered whether his frame could withstand the brutal combat of being an every-down player. His ability to run between the tackles was another concern. But LT is among those select few athletes who, when someone doubts them, don't rest until they prove the doubter wrong.

With solid performances in college all-star games and the NFL Combine, LT had established himself as the best back in the draft—and it didn't take long for the new Charger to make an impact on the NFL. In his first pro game, LT rushed for more than 100 yards. And when the final whistle blew on his rookie season, LT had stuffed his stat sheet with 1,236 rushing yards, 59 catches for 367 receiving yards, and 10 touchdowns—showing the doubters that his 5'10", 221-pound frame could handle the punishment of the marathon NFL season.

LT's career has been nothing short of amazing. From 2001 to 2007, he had seven consecutive 1,000-yard rushing seasons. In 2003, he was the first player in NFL history to rack up 100 receptions and 1,000 rushing yards. He holds NFL single-season records for rushing touchdowns [28], total touchdowns [31], and points scored [186]. He's been named to the Pro Bowl five times, and in 2006 he was named the NFL's Most Valuable Player.

Witnessing LT run up such eye-popping stats on Sunday afternoons season after season might spoil casual fans. But what they don't fully understand is that the ability to post those numbers is created during the off-season, when LT puts unprecedented time and passion into a grueling training program. With strength and conditioning coach Todd Durkin by his side, LT pushes through intense functional sports performance training one day, and follows it with speed, agility, and quickness sessions the next—all to achieve his goal of becoming the best player ever to strap on the pads.

Durkin's Training Goals for LT

Here, Durkin elaborates on LT's training goals, then hits on key points about the workout and the athlete.

Weeks 1-4
1. Establish joint integrity/joint tensile strength
2. Establish foundational strength [balance and core]
3. Improve flexibility [active release technique and PNF stretching]
4. Improve balance in the body [accelerators vs. decelerators; posture; synergistic/ antagonistic]

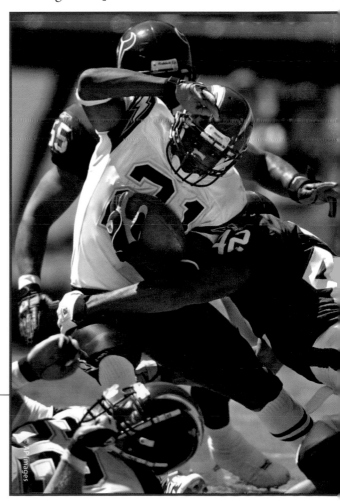

5. Improve functional strength capabilities
6. Establish sound nutritional habits

Weeks 5-10
1. Advance balance and core strength
2. Advance joint integrity
3. Implement specific speed, agility, and explosive drills
4. Advance specific, fundamental functional strength exercises

Weeks 11-16
1. Advance functional strength exercises specific to LT's needs
2. Advance agility, speed, and explosive techniques
3. Follow flexibility and regeneration

principles [massage and bodywork]
4. Do advanced fieldwork to simulate game situations [running, cutting, hopping, jumping, slashing with harnesses, parachutes, bungee cords, vests, etc.]

Important Points About LT's Training and LT Himself

Training Points
1. We do a lot of barefoot work during balance exercises. It strengthens the plantar aponeuroses, ankles, calves and lower shank, which is important for balance and speed.
2. We don't lift a lot of weights; he gets that at the Chargers' Complex. I am big into

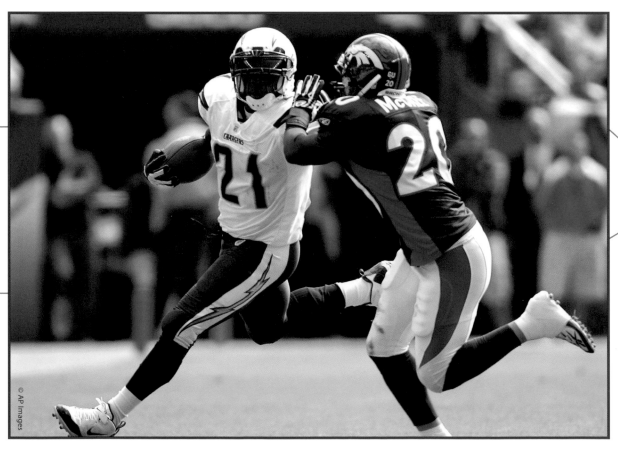

© AP Images

the core, joint integrity, speed, agility, and functional strength with rotation. We do everything with three different foot positions and three different hand positions.

3. We try to use 25-second rests between a lot of our sets, 45 seconds between exercises and about two minutes between modules. It is best to try to simulate game situations.

4. Joint integrity is crucial for us. I want LaDainian to have as much balance and symmetry among his muscles as possible. Our joint integrity program is designed to focus on his feet and ankles, knees, hips and groin, core, shoulders, elbows, and wrists. The program doesn't guarantee that an athlete will be 100 percent injury-proof, but it sure cuts down the likelihood of being injured—especially when you are a running back in the NFL and your body is being abused every week.

5. Rest and rejuvenation are critical. They allow his body to regenerate, and regeneration is a critical phase of the training program.

6. We spend a good deal of time stretching at the end of every workout. Flexibility is critical for LT. We do manual stretching and a type of hands-on bodywork I created, called "Optimal Performance Bodywork." It combines myofasical release, rolling, deep tissue massage, Feldenkrais, and other forms of stretching. We stretch his entire body very well after all workouts.

7. LT receives regular massage and bodywork. I do all of his structural work and fascial work, but he has a few other therapists too. Rob Latimer is a massage therapist who has worked with him for a while. He does a great job helping LT's body, relaxing him,

flushing out soreness, and providing a great overall therapeutic session to help his body recover more quickly.

8. We do a lot of field work as the season approaches. This is where LT needs to be as a running back; he needs to take his hard-earned efforts from the weight room onto the field.

9. When in the weight room, I train LT in an 8' x 8' open space the entire time. I don't need a lot of fancy machines to make him work. We use dumbbells, medicine balls, SPRI cords and bands, balance implements such as Bosu balls, Airex pads, and Dyna discs, and my Keiser equipment. We also do some overspeed training on the Woodway treadmills occasionally. But you would be shocked to learn how much we get done and how hard he works without touching a machine. The machines are a gravy train for us. He has brought in friends, buddies and former college teammates several times to train with him, and they bow out within 20 to 30 minutes because of the intensity.

10. Nutrition is critical, and LT does a great job with his nutritional intake.

11. He often does his speed work wearing an X-Vest.

12. We get in the weight room twice a week and on the field once or twice a week. This is in addition to his reporting two times a week to the Chargers facility for weight training.

LT Points

1. LT is a guy who will outwork anyone. I actually have to put the brakes on him sometimes. He's running hills, doing push-ups and sit-ups all the time, running the

steps in his own home for 30 minutes. He doesn't miss a workout and he's never late for a workout. He's a machine. I have had to monitor him closely so he doesn't overtrain, which can lead to injury.

2. LT loves Walter Payton. He has the same work ethic. LT wants to be the best running back of all time, and that is what drives him to work out like a madman. He highly emulates and respects Emmitt Smith and Barry Sanders, and he loves Walter's heart and passion. That's scary!

3. You will not find a harder worker, or a more dedicated, more committed athlete out there than LaDainian. Everything he gets,

he deserves. He serves the community, signs every autograph, and is thankful and appreciative for all the opportunities God gave him.

4. LT is truly a once-in-a-lifetime athlete, who blends unbelievable talent, extraordinary work ethic, a humble attitude, the willingness to be open minded and learn new information and techniques to help his training, and the grit and determination to be the best running back to ever walk, or run, on this planet.

5. He finished his college degree because he promised his mother he would do it. Relentless!

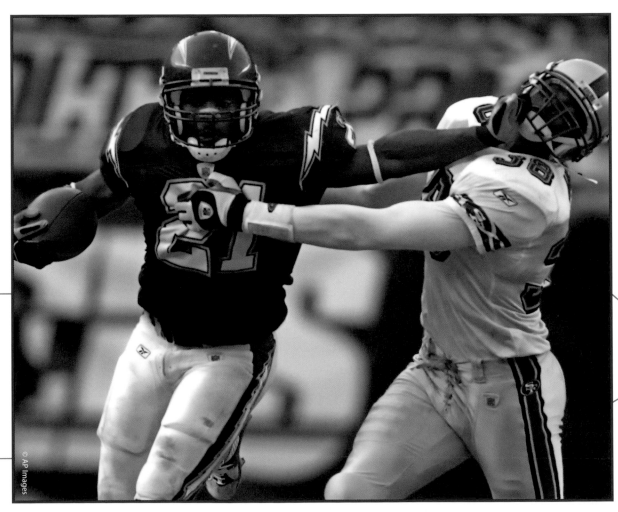

© AP Images

EXERCISES

OVER/UNDER THE FENCE

- Begin in athletic stance with feet shoulder-width apart

- Lift right knee as high as possible; step laterally with right leg and follow with left leg

- Step laterally with right leg under; squat down and duck under an imaginary line; step left leg through

- Repeat pattern in continuous motion for specified reps; perform in opposite direction

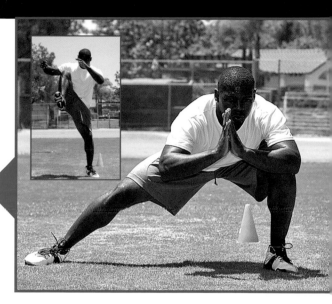

COACHING POINTS

➡ Keep head and chest up throughout exercise ➡ Make sure to imagine stepping over and under fence during each movement ➡ Squat as low as possible when going under fence

BACKWARD LUNGE AND ROTATE

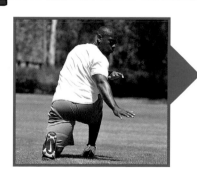

- Step backward with left foot into lunge position

- Twist torso over front leg by taking left elbow to outside of right knee

- Reverse twist back to neutral, returning to start position

- Perform same movement with opposite leg

- Repeat for specified reps

COACHING POINTS

➡ Keep back flat and chest and head up ➡ Do not let front knee slide past foot
➡ Do not let front foot touch ground when stepping into next lunge

3 JOHN TRAVOLTA

- Holding light dumbbells, assume shoulder-width stance on discs

- Raise arms to shoulder level at sides and bend elbows 90 degrees with palms facing forward

- Bring right hand down toward left hip; return to start position

- Perform with opposite hand; repeat for specified reps

COACHING POINTS

- ➧ Keep shoulder blades pinched throughout exercise
- ➧ Do not let stationary arm drop when performing with opposite hand
- ➧ Maintain balance throughout exercise

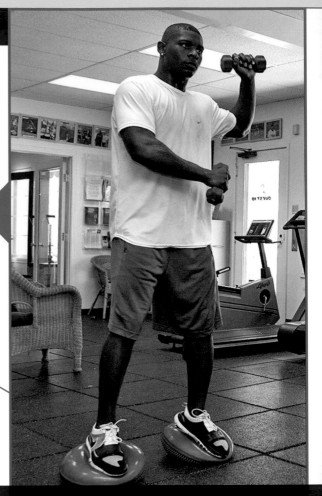

4 BALANCE REACH FORWARD OVER GOAL LINE

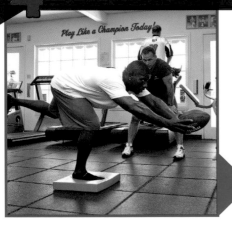

Perform without shoes

- Holding football with both hands, stand on right leg on balance pad with knee slightly flexed

- Fully extend arms and lean forward until back is parallel to ground

- Hold for one second; return to start position

- Repeat for specified reps; switch legs; repeat

COACHING POINTS

- ➧ Draw in abs during exercise
- ➧ Maintain balance throughout exercise
- ➧ Keep head up and back straight

BALANCE SINGLE-LEG 3-POINT TOUCHES

Perform without shoes

- Holding football with both hands, begin with right foot on balance pad in single-leg squat

- Touch toe of left foot to front as far as possible

- Touch toe of left foot to back as far as possible

- Touch toe of left foot to side as far as possible

- Return to start position; repeat for specified reps

- Repeat on opposite leg

COACHING POINTS

- ➡ Keep head up throughout exercise
- ➡ Maintain balance throughout movements
- ➡ Fully extend leg when touching toe to ground

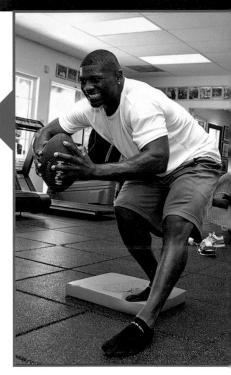

SINGLE-LEG BALANCE ON BOSU AND SIDELINE CATCH DRILL

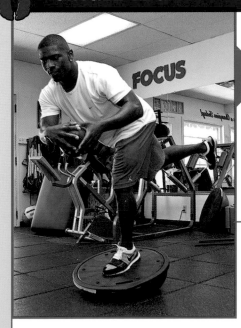

- Balance on left leg on Bosu

- Catch pass from partner five to 10 yards away who is facing shoulder of down leg

- Throw ball back to partner

- Perform for specified reps; repeat on opposite leg

COACHING POINTS

- ➡ Maintain balance and keep core tight throughout exercise
- ➡ Keep head and chest up and back straight
- ➡ Have partner throw catchable balls toward shoulder of down leg

1 JACKKNIFE

- Assume push-up position

- Bring feet toward hands

- Return to start position

- Repeat for specified reps

Coaching Points

- ➤ Keep legs as straight as possible
- ➤ Raise hips when bringing feet toward hands

2 PUSH-UP

- Assume push-up position

- Perform push-ups for specified reps

Coaching Points

- ➤ Keep core tight and legs straight
- ➤ Maintain balance throughout exercise

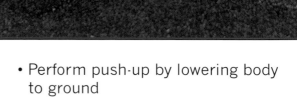

3 JACKKNIFE AND PUSH-UP

- Assume push-up position

- Bring feet toward hands

- Return to start position

- Perform push-up by lowering body to ground

- Explode up to start position

- Repeat for specified reps

Coaching Points

- ➤ Raise hips when bringing feet toward hands
- ➤ Keep core tight and legs straight
- ➤ Maintain balance throughout exercise

CHOPS

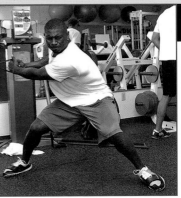
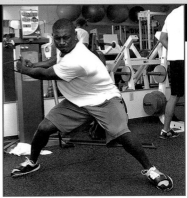

Perform on Keiser or cable machine

Baseball Chop

• With cable machine to right, assume athletic stance with feet slightly wider than shoulder width

• Reach across body with left hand, turning hips and shoulders to cable machine, and hold handle with both hands set at waist height

• Explosively rotate hips left, bringing handle across body until arms are fully extended in front of waist

• Return to start position; repeat for specified reps

• Perform set on opposite side

COACHING POINTS

➡ Turn shoulders toward and away from cable machine with each rep

➡ Make sure hips are pointed away from weight stack at the end of each rep

Low Chop

• With cable machine to right, assume athletic stance with feet slightly wider than shoulder width

• Reach across body with left hand, turning hips and shoulders to cable machine, and hold handle with both hands set at low position

• Explosively rotate hips left, bringing handle across body until above and outside left shoulder

• Return to start position; repeat for specified reps

• Perform set on opposite side

High Chop

• With cable machine to right, assume athletic stance with feet slightly wider than shoulder width

• Reach across body with left hand, turning hips and shoulders to cable machine, and hold handle with both hands set at high position

• Explosively rotate hips left, bringing handle down across body until by left knee

• Return to start position; repeat for specified reps

• Perform set on opposite side

AIR RUNNER SPRINTS

- Assume position in Keiser Air Runner

- Set 40-yard distance on machine

- Perform full speed sprint

- Repeat for specified sets

COACHING POINTS

➡ Keep hips under body and work on acceleration and power

➡ Keep head up throughout exercise

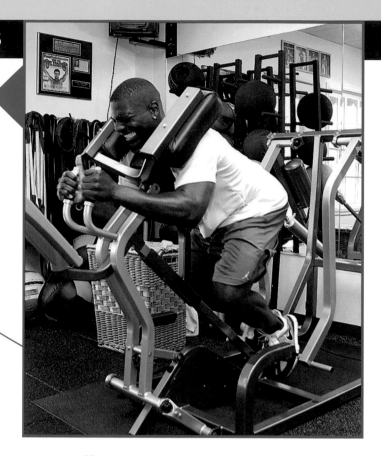

AIR RUNNER LEAP FROGS

- Assume position in Keiser Air Runner

- Explosively jump for specified reps

COACHING POINTS

➡ Exercise should feel like squat jump

➡ Keep head up throughout exercise and perform jumps in continuous fashion

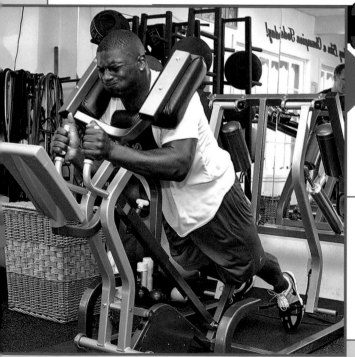

4 CIRCLE DRILL

- Set up three cones in a row three to four yards apart

- Holding football in one hand, sprint to first cone and circle around it

- Repeat to second and third cones

COACHING POINTS

➡ **Perform drill in linear fashion**
➡ **Always face forward when circling**
➡ **Keep head up and body low throughout exercise**

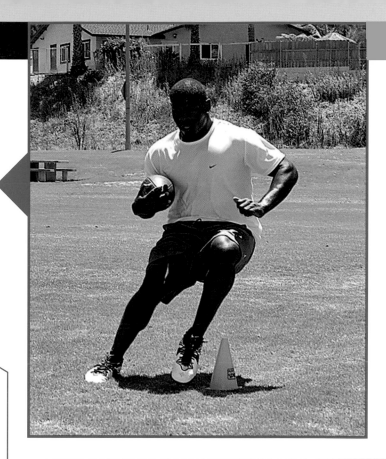

5 OVERSPEED BUNGEE CORD SPRINTS

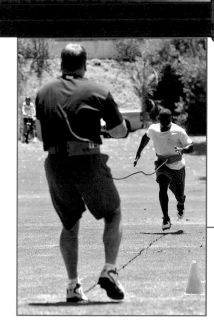

- Begin on line in athletic stance with cord attached to waist and partner holding opposite end in front.

- Run 20 yards with partner pulling in direction of sprint

- Repeat for specified sets

COACHING POINTS

➡ **Maintain slight forward lean**
➡ **Avoid running so hard that you lose form**
➡ **Develop "narrow hallway"—one inch outside of hips and one inch outside of shoulders**
➡ **Avoid swinging arms across body**
➡ **Don't allow feet to swing out to sides**
➡ **Do not open up knees outside of "hallway"**

LT'S TRAINING GUIDE

DAY 1

WARM UP

EXERCISE	SETS/YARDS
High-Knees	1 X 10
Buttkick	1 X 10
A and B Skips	1 X 10
Carioca	1 X 10
Side Run With Leg Crossover	1 X 10
Over/Under the Fence	1 X 10
Frankensteins	1 X 10
Monster Walks	1 X 10
Lunge and Rotate	1 X 10
Backward Lunge and Rotate	1 X 10

STATIONARY

EXERCISE	SETS/REPS
Seal Jacks	1 X 10
Flings	1 X 10
Gate Swings	1 X 10
Pogo Hops	1 X 10
Bodyweight Squats	1 X 10
Side Lunges	1 X 10
Reverse Lunges	1 X 10
Scorpion Kicks	1 X 10
One-Legged Windshield Wipers	1 X 10

BODYWEIGHT

EXERCISE	SETS/REPS
Dirty Dogs	1 X 15
Horseback Riding	1 X 10 each leg on horse, 1 X 10 each leg off horse
45-Degree Straight Leg Extension	1 X 15 each leg
Bird Dog and Rotate	1 X 15 each side
3-Way Push-Ups	1 X 15 each way
Side-Ups With Rotation	1 X 15 each side
Push-Ups With Rotation	1 X 5 each side
PB Horizontal Pull-Ups [4 hand positions]	1 X 8 each way
Side Squat	1 X 15 each way

CORDS OR LIGHT DUMBBELLS

EXERCISE	SETS/REPS
John Travolta	1 X 10 each way
Iron Cross	1 X 15 each way
3-Way Standing Row	1 X 5 each way
Shoulder Clock Work [2 hand positions]	1 X 8 each way
Sport Cord Shoulder Internal/External Rotation	1 X 15 each way
Wall Work	1 X 30 seconds each way

BALANCE CONDITIONING

EXERCISE	SETS/REPS
Balance Touch Floor with Hop	1 X 15 each leg
Balance Reach Forward Over Goal Line	1 X 10 each leg
Balance Single-Leg 3-Point Touches	1 X 5 each way
Single-Leg Balance on Bosu and Sideline Catch Drill	1 X 10 each side

CORE CONDITIONING

EXERCISE	SETS/REPS
Physioball Hip Extensions With Manual Resistance	1 X 15
Physioball Crunches	1 X 25
Physioball Lateral Rolls	1 X 16
Bosu Crunch and Kicks	1 X 15 each way
Side-Lying Bosu Sit-Ups With Rotation	1 X 21 with 21 second hold
Power Wheel (Jackknife, Push-Up, Jackknife and Push-Up)	1 X 15 each exercise
Prone Running Man on Physioball and Bench	1 X 20
Prone Running Man With Knee Twist	1 X 20
Physioball Prone Jackknife and Push-Up	1 X 10
Med Ball Rotation Glute/Hamstring Extension	1 X 16
Keiser 3-Plane Wood Chops	1 X 15 each direction

PLYOS

EXERCISE	SETS/REPS
Vertimax Squat Jumps	3 X 10
Lunge Hops With Med Ball Twist	2 X 20
Skater Plyos	2 X 20
Single-Leg Lateral Bounds	2 X 20
Bulgarian Lunge Hops	2 X 20

FOOT QUICKNESS

EXERCISE	SETS/REPS
Hip Disassociation Drill	2 X 10 seconds
2 Bosu High-Knee Drill With Football	2 X 15 seconds
5-Dot Drill With Twist	2 X 20 seconds
Bosu Toe Taps	2 X 15 seconds
Bosu Lateral Hops	2 X 20 seconds

FUNCTIONAL STRENGTH AND POWER

EXERCISE	SETS/REPS
Keiser Air Runner Sprints	3 X 40 yards
Keiser Air Runner Leap Frogs	3 X 12
Multi-Directional Lunges	2 X 20
Straight Leg Deadlifts	2 X 15
Physioball Leg Curls	2 X 15
Physioball Dumbbell Bench Press	3 X 15
Keiser Functional Trainer Single-Arm Row and Rotates	3 X 15

DAY 2

AGILITY: LADDER DRILLS

EXERCISE	SETS/REPS
One Foot in Each	1 X 2
Two Feet in Each	1 X 2
Two In, One Out	1 X 2
Two Out, One In	1 X 2
Lateral Shuffle	1 X 2

AGILITY: CONE DRILLS

EXERCISE	SETS/REPS
Box Drill	1 X 1
Circle Drill	1 X 1
Zigzag Drill	1 X 1

AGILITY: FORM RUNNING

EXERCISE	SETS/REPS
Run With Perfect Form	1 X 5 minutes

AGILITY: RESISTED SPEED RUNNING

EXERCISE	SETS/YARDS
Towing With Harness	6 X 30
Overspeed Bungee Cord Sprints	4 X 20

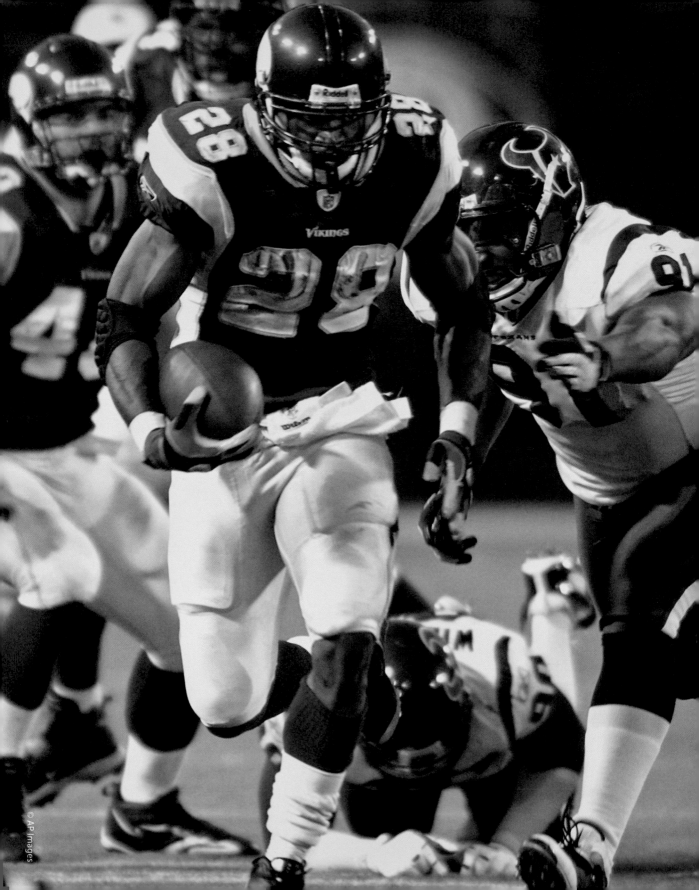

CHAPTER 8

ADRIAN PETERSON

WORKING OUT WITH PATRICK WILLIS AND ALAN BRANCH

EDITOR'S NOTE

Today, Adrian Peterson is a huge NFL star—perhaps the league's best running back. When we caught up with him in February 2007, however, he was a doubted NFL prospect whose draft status was on the verge of plummeting.

During his career at Oklahoma, Peterson's relentless, I'd-rather-die-than-step-out-of-bounds style of running had allowed him to trounce opposing Big 12 defenses and had made him the likely No. 1 overall pick in the 2007 NFL Draft. But all of that hard-nosed running had also taken a toll on Peterson's body. Nagging injuries—including a busted shoulder and a strained knee—had prevented him from reaching his full potential in college. NFL scouts had more than enough reason to question his durability.

Nevertheless, we wanted Peterson on our magazine cover from the moment he turned his attention to the NFL Combine. He had one of the most athletic physiques we'd ever seen, and he trained with the kind of dedication and toughness that defines NFL greats. For those same reasons, he was the perfect athlete to grace the cover of this book.

ADRIAN PETERSON BREAKS LOOSE DURING A GAME AGAINST THE TEXANS IN 2008. PETERSON'S COMBINATION OF POWER AND SPEED MAKE HIM A TOP NFL RUNNING BACK.

When we witnessed his training at Athletes' Performance in Tempe, Arizona, Peterson wasn't quite 100 percent; but nobody could tell. That day, the hungry running back's body looked indestructible and explosive as he ripped through his speed training. A few exercises were modified to relieve the pressure on his knee, but overall he looked ready to pound it between the tackles or to cut outside to take it to the house.

Peterson's mental toughness and daily doses of AP training helped get him back to full health in time for the NFL Combine, where he ran a 4.38-second 40-yard dash—heady stuff for a 6'2", 220-pound power back. His performance at the Combine prevented Peterson from plummeting completely. He did slip to the seventh overall pick, which turned out to be a steal for the Minnesota Vikings.

Taking the draft drop in stride, Peterson immediately established himself as the most explosive back in the NFL, rushing for 1,341 yards and scoring 13 TDs in his rookie season. The following year, he elevated his game even further, leading the league in rushing with 1,760 yards. Two 1,000-yard seasons, two Pro-Bowl nods, and one definitive answer to the question of his durability.

Alongside Peterson during his crucial workouts at AP were two other men looking to crush similar doubts. Patrick Willis had dominated the linebacker position at Ole Miss, winning the Butkus Award his senior season. But the lack of big-time exposure for Ole Miss football left NFL scouts uneasy. At 6'5", 330 pounds, Alan Branch possessed all the necessary tools to be an imposing defensive lineman during his time at Michigan. However, some NFL gurus thought he was a bit lazy and lacked dedication to the game. Willis went on to win the NFC Rookie of the Year Award and is still beating backs to the hole on a regular basis. Branch was a force for the Phoenix Cardinals' defensive line during their 2008 Super Bowl run.

The following is *STACK's* cover feature on Adrian Peterson, Patrick Willis, and Alan Branch, which originally appeared in the April 2007 issue of the magazine.

THE BEST GET BETTER

Lounging around in a semi-circle on the training floor at Athletes' Performance in Tempe, Arizona, is a mind-boggling collection of talent. It's as if some audacious creative director has brought together the most recognizable, gifted college football players in the nation for an epic ad campaign.

Oklahoma's Adrian Peterson is discussing a recent addition to the "Diesel" tattoo carved into his sculpted right shoulder with fellow all-star Patrick Willis, a linebacker from Ole Miss. Alan Branch, the best defensive lineman in the country, is getting loose alongside former Notre Dame quarterback Brady Quinn. The scenario is even more unbelievable because it is not a one-time event created to entertain or inspire. These hungry young men have been side by side every morning for weeks, grooming every aspect of their bodies in hopes of impressing NFL coaches at the Combine and their individual Pro Days.

Luke Richesson, the performance specialist charged with getting these gridiron greats NFL-ready, says, "This has been seven years in the making. We started our first class with one first-rounder; then we got four, then six, and it just went from there. Talent attracts talent, and we've worked hard to step up our game and take our methods to the next level. This has culminated in our having about 30 guys here who have a legitimate shot at having long, successful NFL careers."

The Athletes' Performance phenomenon is not limited to the Tempe, Arizona, facility that Willis, Peterson and Branch currently inhabit. The same star-studded training takes place at AP's Los Angeles, Las Vegas, and Gulf Breeze, Florida, locations. In all of these facilities, the best get even better.

Patrick Willis

Position: LB
College: University of Mississippi
Height: 6'1"
Weight: 240 lbs
Scouting Report: The Butkus Award winner and two-time All-American is the best linebacker in the draft. Willis, who recorded 137 tackles his senior season at Ole Miss, was named the Senior Bowl's Defensive Player of the Game after recording 11 tackles. He plays sideline to sideline, consistently beating backs to the hole with his blazing speed, quickness, and instinct. Willis' maturity, leadership, and respect for coaches and opposing players will make him a positive addition to any defense.

Richesson on Willis: He is very explosive. He may not have known how exactly to express all of that power, but Patrick is an exceptional athlete. After a few verbal cues, he made all the adjustments almost immediately. He may be one of the fastest 240-pound guys we've ever seen. Patrick wanted to improve his flexibility and overall movement, which we've been able to accomplish.

Willis On:

Showing off for NFL coaches: I'm looking forward to impressing some people by testing well in everything. Hopefully, they'll be impressed with my speed.

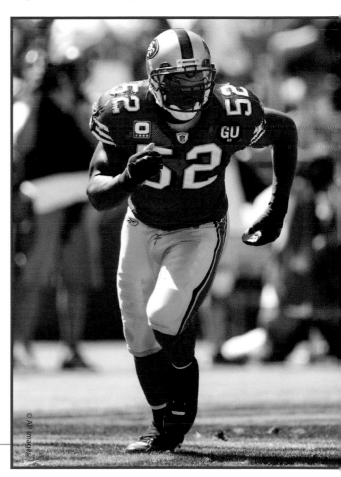

PATRICK WILLIS HEADS UP THE FIELD.

AP's all-star class: To be honest, it's a huge honor to be around these guys every day. Coming from Ole Miss and not getting a lot of exposure, I feel like I'm the one enjoying this the most. I mean, these are the guys I've watched on *SportsCenter* and in big bowl games. I just love waking up every morning, coming in here to watch these guys work out, and then getting to work out with them.

Lining up together: I'd love the opportunity to play alongside these guys.

What drives him: We've all experienced adversity, so to be where we are now is such a blessing. And when something happens now, it doesn't really compare to what we went through to get here. I just take it with a grain of salt and run with it.

The NFL dream: I've wanted to play in the National Football League since I can remember—before I even knew anything about college football. I remember watching the Dallas Cowboys—Jay Novacek, Emmitt Smith, Troy Aikman, and Michael Irvin—and wanting to be like them. Then I was told I had to play college football first, which I didn't even know. I remember thinking, "Alright, whatever it takes to get to that next level."

Being a role model: For the most part, if you do what you are supposed to do and leave a good legacy, then it shouldn't be a problem. Stepping in and becoming a role model should be pretty natural for me.

Adrian Peterson

Position: RB
College: University of Oklahoma
Height: 6'2"
Weight: 220 lbs
Scouting Report: His unbelievable combo of size, speed, and power make Peterson the best running back in the nation. He loves to deliver the blow, but he can also outrun any defender on the field. His balance, patience, and vision have drawn comparisons to the great Eric Dickerson. In his freshman season, Peterson scored 15 touchdowns and set the NCAA's single-season rushing record for a freshman, with 1,925 yards. As a sophomore in 2004, he finished second in the Heisman balloting. Peterson totaled 4,045 career rushing yards in three years—just short of the Oklahoma record, which he would've shattered if injuries hadn't plagued him. He's nicknamed "AD, All Day," because he can run over any defense, all day long.

Richesson on Peterson: Adrian wants to wow people with his speed. And much like Patrick and Alan, he has a lot of raw horsepower. In college, your manhood is tested by how hard you continue to grind and work, and Adrian passed. He's coming off a shoulder injury, so we made sure he stays healthy by continuing to refine his movement skills. He might be one of the fastest running backs in history if he does what we think he's capable of doing.

Peterson On:

Showing off for NFL coaches: I definitely want to show my speed. I've got my technique down, so I am excited about getting out there and running a good 40 for the NFL coaches. I'm excited about the vertical jump, too.

AP's all-star class: Being around all these stars is cool; I really enjoy it. And I don't know what Patrick's talking about—he's a freak, man! We all have different personalities, but the same work ethic and drive, which is cool. It makes you realize how all these guys got to this level.

Lining up together: Oh boy! That would be some all-star team.

What drives him: I definitely have the inspiration and drive I need. I think about all the hard work I've put in since I was seven years old to get to this point. I've been through battles and difficult times; so now at this point, when things get tough, getting through it is nothing.

The NFL dream: Growing up watching Emmitt Smith and Eddie George, I always wanted to be in the National Football League. That was always my ultimate dream. In high school, I went through the process of getting my name out there so I could play in college. Now I'm ready to take that third step.

Being a role model: I'm quite comfortable in the spotlight and being a role model. Like I said, when I was little, I had guys I looked up to and tried to be like. I know how important it is, because kids do what they see on television. Now that I'm in the position where kids out there want to be like me, it feels good to do right and show them how hard work makes an opportunity like this possible.

Alan Branch

Position: DT
College: University of Michigan
Height: 6'6"
Weight: 331 lbs

Scouting Report: The best defensive lineman in the country is huge—great size on a great frame. Branch is extremely strong, and even more impressive is his movement for a big man; he can cover 40 yards in five seconds flat. This allows him to take on multiple blockers and to play virtually every position on the defensive

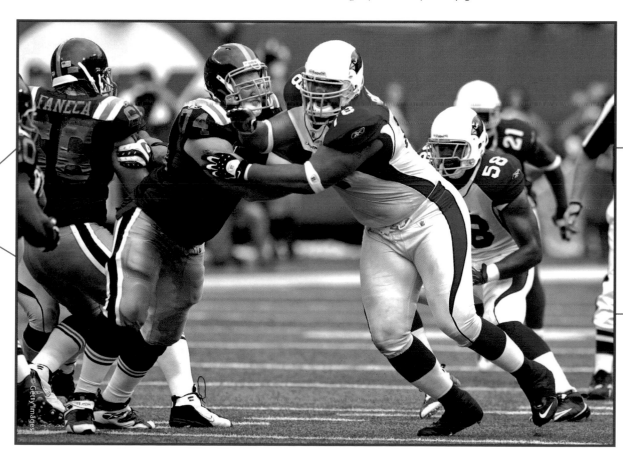

ALAN BRANCH FIGHTS OFF A BLOCK.

line. Branch plays the run better than anyone and delivers punishing blows at the point of contact, often in the backfield. The three-year starter amassed nine sacks and 18 tackles for a loss in his 37 games as a Wolverine.

Richesson on Branch: Obviously, the first thing you notice about Alan is his size. But just from watching him goof around, I could tell he can move. He has this uncanny ability to dance. Not many big guys can do what he can. He's really prospered in our system when it came to movement. He has natural ability, but he needed to know a few finer details. Once he got those, he really improved.

Branch On:

Showing off for NFL coaches: I know I'm not going to shock anyone with my speed like these guys, but I am going out there to show off my athleticism. For as big as I am, not too many people can move like I do.

AP's all-star class: Everybody here is good people, so that's the best part. A lot of us have the same attitude; we are all working hard to get to the same place. It's kind of funny to think that I saw these guys on TV all season, and now I see them face to face, on a more personal level.

Lining up together: That's one of the first things I talked about when I got here. When I saw Patrick's speed, I just imagined having him back there as my linebacker. My linebackers, Dave Harris and Prescott Burgess, were good, but I can just imagine this guy's speed behind me.

What drives him: I just think about all the people who want to be in our position. Rough times happen, but there are a lot more people who want to be here than anywhere else. Knowing that keeps me going.

The NFL dream: It's always been a dream. But to be honest, when I was little, I knew it

was a stretch. Being a kid from New Mexico, I didn't know anyone from there who got to this level, so I was just glad to keep playing when I got to college. I never thought I would get to play for Michigan, which has always been my favorite team. And because I'm my hardest critic, I didn't realize I would be in this position until about three months ago. During the year, I didn't think I was doing well enough to get here, but I was. I just wasn't good enough to please myself.

Being a role model: I've always been the role-model type. When I was growing up, I always worked with younger kids and had fun with them to make sure that they were on the right path toward having a successful future.

Richesson's Plan

Willis, Peterson, and Branch were already tremendous athletes when they showed up on AP's Tempe campus, but Richesson still had work to do to prep them for their NFL auditions—and little time to do it.

"These guys are coming off a very long season, 14 games for some," Richesson says. "The car has been knocked out of alignment so to speak. First we have to get these guys reconditioned, then still make improvements within the six to eight weeks we have. Our main focus is putting them back together while simultaneously pushing the envelope with their strength and power."

AP's use of core, flexibility, and balance work to rebuild the body is new to most football players. Richesson says, "These guys have a hard time believing how easy the workouts are for them. Don't get me wrong. We push them, but with more of a focus on quality, not quantity. They've proven they have strength and power to battle the entirety of a game, so we focus on the finer points."

All three future NFL stars have embraced AP's "finer-points" approach. "This training is so much more specific and hands-on than what I'm used to," Peterson says. "We work on all the small things, which is a little different for me, too."

For Willis, the training has resulted in improved flexibility. He says, "The flexibility allows me to run a little bit faster and move a little better than I did. A lot of it has to do with the work we've done on my hips—much more than I was used to, but it's all part of the core and flexibility work they stress here."

Branch's body has slimmed down 10 pounds so far, but he says, "that isn't the biggest response my body has had to this training. I've really improved my flexibility and balance more than I thought possible."

Richesson says this about the workout Peterson, Willis, and Branch are performing this particular day: "Everything about it is geared toward the explosion and power needed for a good 40. There's no way around it; everything is based on those 40 yards, and even the first 10 yards of explosion."

And so begins the journey to a blazing 40 and NFL stardom.

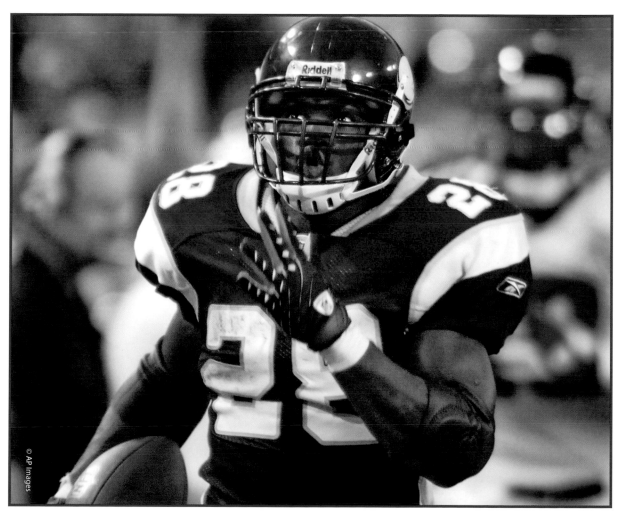

© AP Images

DYNAMIC WARM-UP

Richesson: This specific warm-up focuses on increasing hip separation and mobility. The larger the range of motion of their strides, the more power they can put into the ground.

LUNGE WITH ELBOW TO INSTEP AND EXTENSION

- Step forward with right foot into lunge

- Lower chest until right forearm touches floor to inside of right foot

- Straighten right leg

- Repeat with left leg

Benefits: Enhances flexibility in hips, hamstrings, lower back, torso, groin and hip flexors

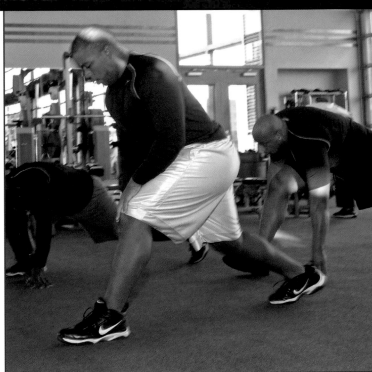

COACHING POINTS

Use forearm for support if necessary
Extend leg as far as possible
Avoid stretching to point of pain

2 INCHWORM

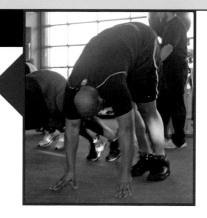

- Beginning in push-up position, walk feet toward hands, keeping legs straight

- Walk hands out until back in push-up position

- Repeat

Benefits: Strengthens and lengthens muscles // Loosens hamstrings, glutes and lower back // Prevents muscle tears and pulls

COACHING POINTS

- ➤ Make sure all muscles go through full range of motion
- ➤ Do not strain muscles
- ➤ Do not take big steps with feet or hands

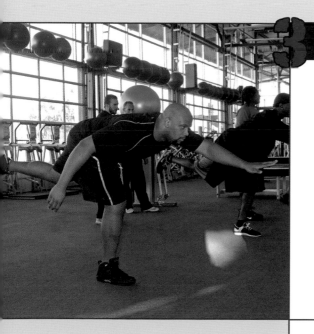

3 SINGLE-LEG ANTERIOR REACH

- Standing on right foot, bend at waist so chest is parallel to ground

- Extend left leg back and right arm forward; hold

- Repeat on left leg

Benefits: Works single-leg strength and balance // Stretches and lengthens muscles

COACHING POINTS

- ➤ Keep leg straight
- ➤ Maintain balance
- ➤ Focus on body being parallel to ground

STRAIGHT-LEG MARCH

4

- Keeping legs straight, kick them one at a time up to shoulder level

- Continue in walking fashion

Benefits: Gets the blood flowing before a workout // Improves flexibility

COACHING POINTS

➼ Keep kicking leg straight
➼ Raise leg as high as possible
➼ Use slow, controlled movements

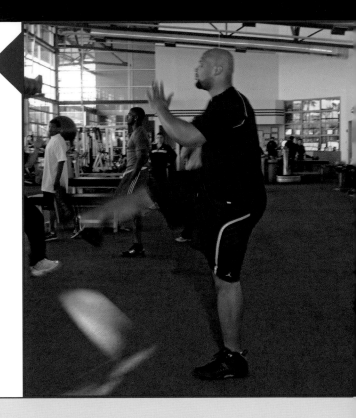

HIGH-KNEE MARCH

5

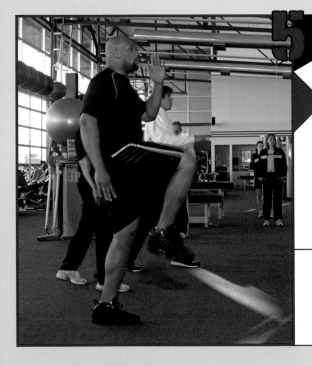

- Perform high knees in slow, controlled manner, holding each high-knee position for one full second

Benefits: Gets the blood flowing before workout // Creates mobility in joints and hips

COACHING POINTS

➼ Lift knee as high as possible
➼ Avoid swinging leg too much
➼ Use slow, controlled movements

POWER CIRCUIT

Richesson: Once we've improved hip range of motion and stride length with the warm-up, we work on putting power into the ground. This simulates the first steps of the 40, and it helps them become as explosive as possible with those steps. We hold the bottom position [of the squat], because in the 40, they have to explode out of a completely static, stopped position with the front leg.

SINGLE-LEG BUNGEE-RESISTED SQUAT

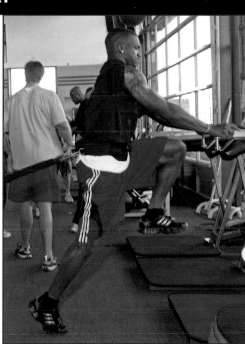

- Attach bungee cord to waist as partner holds it from behind you to apply tension

- Balance on right leg and keep left foot elevated behind you

- Drive hips back and squat down

- Keeping right knee directly above foot, hold low position for full second

- Explode forward and up, driving left knee up until you reach full extension with right leg

- Hold extended position for full second; repeat for specified reps

- Perform set on opposite side

Benefits: Improves putting power into the ground // Simulates first steps of the 40, helping athlete become as explosive as possible with first steps // Holding the bottom position helps an athlete explode out of completely static, stopped position with the front leg

COACHING POINTS

➤ Keep good posture, and focus on getting full hip extension at the top

➤ As you lower, make sure to keep your knee over your foot so you have a good angle from which to drive

Richesson: It's a dynamic, active isolation stretch. Symmetry within an athlete is important; so if one side is tighter than the other, focus on that side a little more.

- Lie on stomach on training table

- Keeping abdomen and hips against table, assist as partner raises your right heel toward your butt

- Partner applies pressure at point of tension for one second; relax

- Repeat for specified reps

- Perform set on opposite leg

Benefits: Increases flexibility in the quad and hip flexors

COACHING POINTS

➡ Avoid stretching past point of pain
➡ Hold position until well stretched

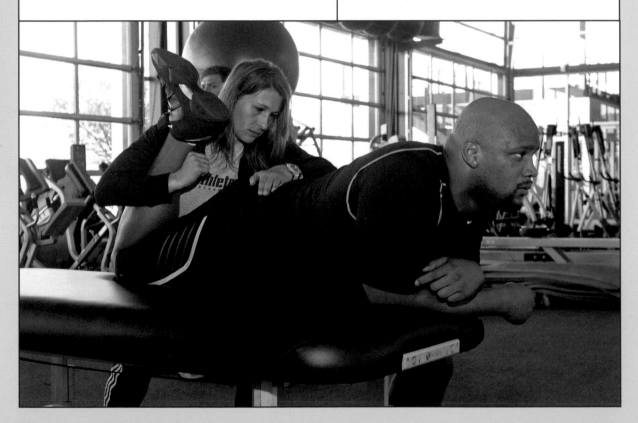

3 PHYSIOBALL LEG RAISE

Richesson: In absolute speed, you need strength to hold the proper sprinting posture. A lot of guys are weak [in the hip flexors and lower abdominals], so they break down after 20 yards.

- Lie with lower back on physioball, holding onto stable object behind head

- Keeping legs bent 90 degrees, lower them with control until feet nearly touch floor

- Raise legs and curl body to bring knees above chest

- Repeat for specified reps

Benefits: Strengthens hip flexors and lower abdominals

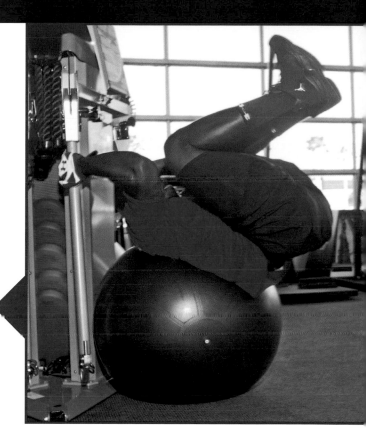

COACHING POINTS

➡ Keep movement slow and controlled to avoid relying on momentum

SPEED WORK

EXPLOSIVE STARTS

Richesson: This [speed] progression is based on stability; we are trying to give them the ability to hold that posture. We want them to be able to generate power from that loaded position. If they can't hold the single-leg position, they will greatly limit their explosion.

- Assume single-leg stance with forward body lean and off leg elevated behind

- Bend balancing knee; hold position for full second

- Keeping head down and chest low, explode out by driving off leg

- Stay low and accelerate for 15 yards

- After three reps on each leg, perform three 40 starts

Benefits: Generates power from a stable, loaded position // Develops single-leg strength, which creates explosion

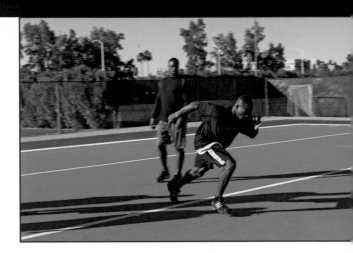

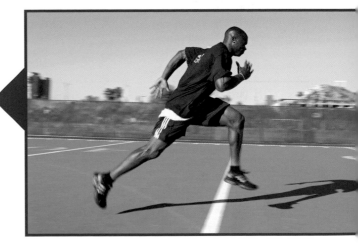

COACHING POINTS

- ➡ Load front leg by pressing heel into ground
- ➡ Keep head down and focus on quick, powerful arm swings

ADRIAN PETERSON'S TRAINING GUIDE

DYNAMIC WARM-UP

Lunge With Elbow to Instep and Extension

Inchworm

Single-Leg Anterior Reach

Straight-Leg March

High-Knee March

*Perform each dynamic exercise over 10 yards; repeat.

POWER CIRCUIT

	SETS	REPS
Single-Leg Bungee-Resisted Squat	2	3 each leg
Partner Quad/Hip Flexor Stretch	3	8-10 each leg
Physioball Leg Raise	3	10-15

*Perform all three exercises as a circuit; rest after completing full cycle.

SPEED WORK

	SETS	REPS
Explosive Starts	1	3 each leg
40-Yard dash	1	3

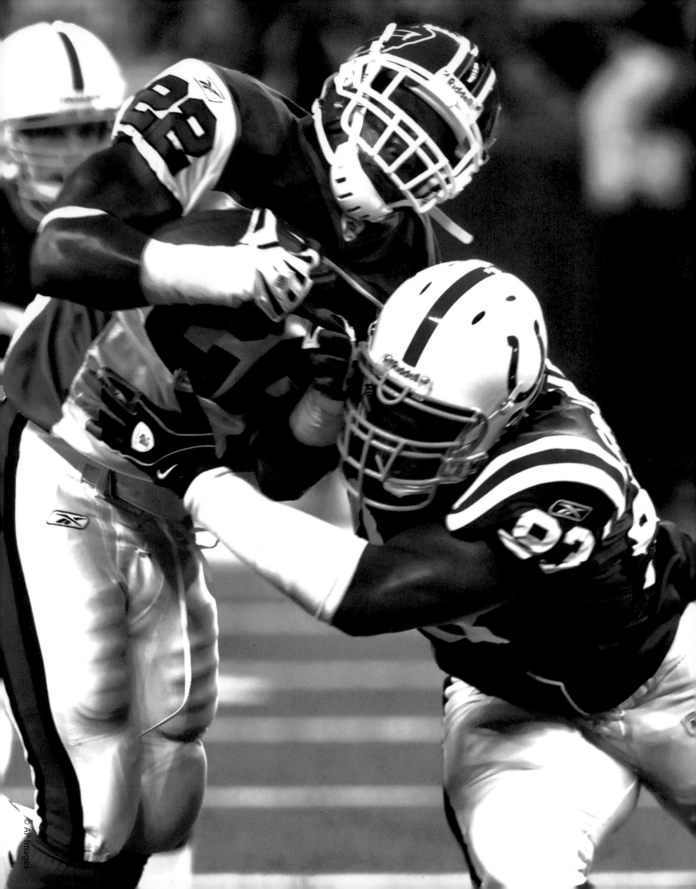

CHAPTER 9

DWIGHT FREENEY

EDITOR'S NOTE

We conducted our training and cover shoot with Pro Bowl defensive end Dwight Freeney at the legendary Gold's Gym in Venice Beach, California, in the early summer of 2008. At that time, the 6'1", 280-plus-pounder was still recovering from the debilitating foot injury that prematurely ended his '07 NFL campaign. Some questioned whether he could return to his high-caliber style of play during the 2008 season and beyond, but we had faith in Freeney's determination to get back on the field. Still, since he was slated to begin camp on the Physically Unable to Perform List, we assumed his training would be a pretty casual affair. We were wrong.

Freeney is a massive man, full of well-shaped muscles. His size was a real surprise to us, because he has made his name as an explosive, athletic DE, one who plays a couple of speeds faster than other NFL linemen. His 70.5 career sacks suddenly made more sense.

The moment he walked through the door at Gold's, Freeney caught the eye of every spandex-clad muscleman in the gym. But those bodybuilders, with their tanned, veiny, compact balls of muscle, weren't sizing up the Colts star as one of their own. On the contrary, they were

DWIGHT FREENEY HITS FRED JACKSON OF THE BILLS DURING A GAME IN 2008. FREENEY'S AMAZING CORE STRENGTH IS A KEY TO HIS SUCCESS AS A PASS RUSHER.

all suddenly afflicted with serious self-consciousness. As Freeney made his way across the main training floor, a sea of people in denim cutoffs, tank tops, and work boots parted for the only real athlete in the building. Most eyes quickly found the ground as humiliation set in.

Behind the NFL's best pass rusher walked William Hicks, Freeney's college strength coach from Syracuse. Hicks was excited to show us what Freeney can do in the weight room, work that enables him to dominate quarterbacks at a ridiculous level—for example, his league-leading 16 sacks in 2004. Coach Hicks put Freeney through an incredibly demanding, non-stop upper-body strength workout. The goal was to increase the power of Freeney's already-punishing punches, swipes, and swims, while also improving his conditioning with short rest periods.

We were wrong about the intensity of his workout, but right in believing in Freeney's rapid return to the gridiron. Later that summer, he completed his recovery and bounced back to his prior form for the Colts. During the 2008 season, he drove rival QBs into the ground 10.5 times, made 24 solo tackles, and earned another trip to Hawaii. Opposing offensive linemen should be very afraid of what this guy will be able to do after a full off-season of training.

Here is the article from the October 2009 issue of *STACK* Magazine.

QUARTERBACK ASSASSIN

A defensive end's pass rushing responsibility is to get to the quarterback as quickly as possible. Sounds easy, right? Now insert an athletic 320-pound tackle and a nimble 220-pound running back to help block. The destructive path to that quick release, fleet-footed quarterback is severely hindered—unless you're Dwight Freeney. Freeney's strength and perseverance have made him into one of the league's most consistent quarterback assassins.

Over the past eight seasons with the Indianapolis Colts, defensive end Dwight Freeney has been a quarterback's worst nightmare. A four-time Pro Bowler and Super Bowl XLI champ, Freeney was the AFC's Defensive Player of the Year in 2005. He is the Colts' all-time sacks leader with 70.5—a stat that puts him in an elite pass-rushing club. Considering that at 6'1" and 268 pounds, Freeney is regarded as undersized for a defensive end, his achievements are even more impressive.

When Freeney came out of high school in Connecticut, college recruiters knew he could be an impact player, but as a linebacker or a tight end—not a prolific pass rusher. Yet with his unwavering passion, Freeney forged his reputation by putting signal-callers on their backs.

"I started getting letters my junior year from schools," he says. "Then when I went on a visit they would say, 'We don't want you to play defensive end; we want you to play linebacker.' Or, 'You're not as tall as we thought you were going to be, and we don't want you anymore.' I used all that as motivation.

"It's about how hard you play and making plays on the field," he continues. "At some point, somebody's going to have to recognize it—and if they don't, just keep on doing it."

Fortunately, a few schools recognized Freeney's potential as a destructive end, so he had options with his college choice. He decided on Syracuse University, where he proceeded to wreak havoc on opposing Big East backfields. "Syracuse was a perfect fit for me," Freeney says. "It was close enough to home, where I could go home, [but] far enough away, too. When I was choosing a school, it was important [to me that] they had a great history. The legends that have gone there—like Jim Brown, Floyd Little, Larry Csonka, Donovan McNabb, and Marvin Harrison—that was big for me."

It's safe to assume that Freeney is also considered an Orange legend. During his senior season, he set a school record with 17.5 sacks, ending his career with 34—second all-time in 'Cuse history. He also set an NCAA single-season record for forced fumbles [8] and fumble recoveries [3]. A consensus All-American, he was a finalist for the Lombardi [best lineman], Bednarik [top defensive player], and Nagurski [outstanding defensive player] awards. Combined, Freeney's stats and accolades silenced the critics and convinced the Colts to draft him 11th overall in the 2002 NFL Draft, making his dream a reality.

"I definitely dreamt of being a professional athlete while I looked up to Lawrence Taylor," he says. "I loved how he was relentless playing the game from sideline to sideline."

Although he may not be on Taylor's level quite yet, Freeney has NFL offensive coordinators plotting to frustrate his constant QB harassment. With superhuman strength and

a deadly arsenal of moves, he will continue to be an unwelcome visitor in opponents' backfields. "My favorite thing to do on the field is hitting the quarterback," Freeney says. "It doesn't matter [how I get to the quarterback]—I could cartwheel or backflip, I could get thrown into him—there's no bad move. I'll get to him using speed, power, or spinning, just as long as I'm hitting him. That's the best thing in the world."

To maintain his toughness, this hard-hitting sack master hits the weights hard during the off-season, part of which he spends with his former strength and conditioning coach at Syracuse, William Hicks. The two have spent 10 years together, sculpting Freeney into the player he is today. "[Hicks has] trained a lot of guys that

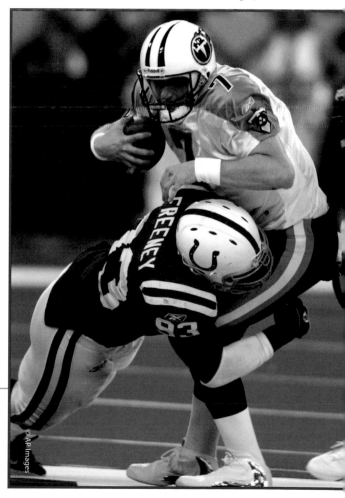

have played in the [NFL], and he understands what I need," Freeney says. "No matter what we're doing, he keeps it fresh and interesting. We're not doing the same stuff all the time, and he knows how to push me."

According to Hicks, the two have mutual respect for each other's talents. "Dwight's not going to do the same thing every day and get in a rut," Hicks says. "He wants me to challenge him in such a way that the workout pushes him past where he went the [time] before."

From 2002 to 2005, grit and determination helped Freeney notch four consecutive double-digit sack seasons. But he was sub-par in '06, with 5.5 sacks; and in 2007, he was sidelined with a foot injury, lacing up for only nine games. Looking to regain his dominance, Freeney took his aggression out during the off-season, coming back with 10.5 sacks in 2008.

Hicks stresses that football-specific training is a focus of every workout, and it played a key role in helping Freeney recover from his injury—to be better than ever. "You really want to make sure that you work the energy system that's going to be played in the game," Hicks says. "Football is more of an anaerobic sport than an aerobic sport, so we set up the rest time to mimic the game. As far as doing reps, everything Dwight does is in an explosive manner. Sports are played with power, not necessarily strength."

Freeney adds, "I want to build as much muscle and as much endurance as I can to get my body as fine-tuned as possible. During the season, you're not going to be able to have those opportunities to really continue that, and your muscles are going to break down. It's a long year, so you want to build up as much as possible and get your body in the best shape to endure the long season."

Monday workouts focus on the muscles that help Freeney push and punch [chest, shoulders, and triceps]—essential to helping him gain the explosive strength needed to get by bigger tackles. "To best utilize what his talents are, we have to train explosively. And if we train slow, like a bodybuilder, we won't utilize what he brings to the table," Hicks says. "Today we were

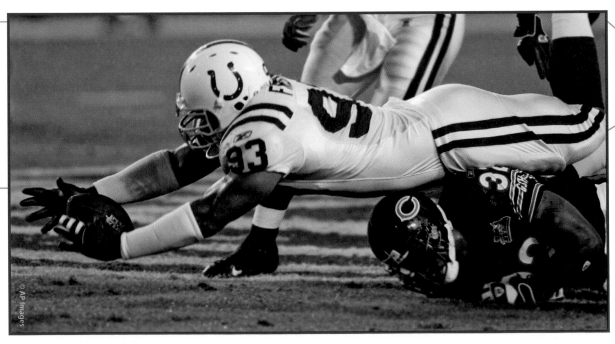

© AP Images

working on his primary movers in his upper body, which deliver his punch and push against opponents. We're also focusing on his main source of power, his core. We're big believers in training from the belly button out."

When an athlete and a coach are dedicated to and believe in the same philosophy as much as Freeney and Hicks do, special things happen. "Our workouts are so explosive and core-heavy, [which] really benefit me on the field, because it's one exercise right after another with minimal rest—and that's what I need," Freeney says. "My body responds very well to this, and I can get in shape pretty fast with this type of workout. We like to do more explosive work, because it gets me ready faster."

With dedication and work ethic that are second to none, Freeney proves he could have been just as dominant in the NFL as a linebacker or tight end.

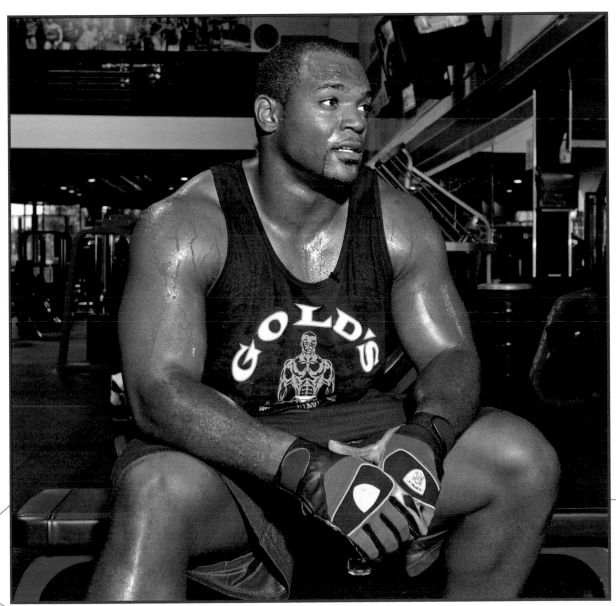

CORE WARM-UP

TOE TOUCHES

Hicks: Basically, what you're doing is working your core strength, but at the same time putting the hamstring in a pre-stretched position.

- Lie with back on ground and legs straight up toward ceiling

- Keeping arms straight, crunch up until fingertips touch toes

- Lower with control; repeat for specified reps

COACHING POINTS

➤ Keep legs as straight as possible and toes pulled back

➤ Legs should form 90-degree angle from ground

➤ Keep back flat and head in neutral position

➤ Avoid using body for momentum

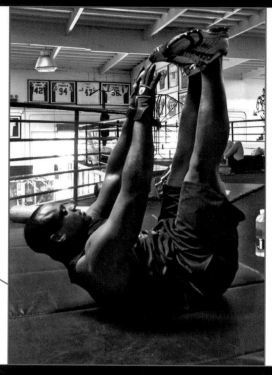

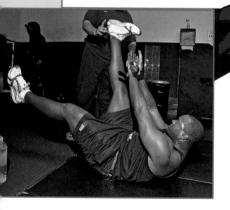

SINGLE-LEG TOE TOUCHES

Hicks: This has the same benefits as the toe touches, but it brings more of the hip flexor into play.

- Lie with back on ground and legs up in scissor position

- Keeping arms straight, crunch up until fingertips touch toes of elevated foot

- Lower with control; repeat for specified reps

- Perform set with opposite leg raised

COACHING POINTS

➤ Keep one leg up, 90 degrees from ground, and opposite leg bent 45 degrees on ground

➤ Keep core tight and maintain good posture throughout exercise

➤ Keep back flat and head in neutral position

➤ Avoid using body for momentum

3 SINGLE-LEG REACH THROUGH

Hicks: He's going to get a little more flexibility with this exercise, since he has to reach his hands toward the leg that's on the ground.

- Lie with back on ground and legs up in scissor position

- Keeping arms straight, crunch up and forward toward foot of lower leg

- Lower with control; repeat for specified reps

- Perform set with opposite leg raised

COACHING POINTS

- ➤ Keep one leg up, 90 degrees from ground, and opposite leg bent 45 degrees on ground
- ➤ Keep core tight and maintain good posture throughout exercise
- ➤ Keep back flat and head in neutral position
- ➤ Avoid using body for momentum

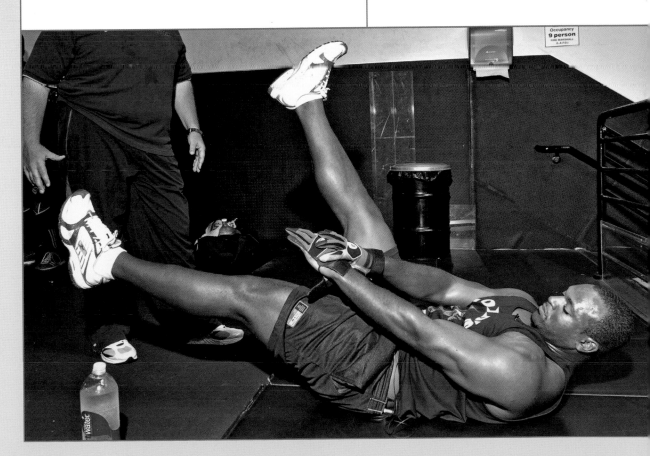

4 FULL SIT-UP

Hicks: Performing the full sit-up really brings into play the hip flexors, quads, low back and abs.

- Assume sit-up position with feet flat on ground

- Without rocking, perform sit-up

- Lower slowly until shoulder blades reach floor

- Repeat for specified reps

COACHING POINTS

- ➡ Place hands on ears and keep elbows back and feet flat on floor
- ➡ Pull body up through belly button
- ➡ Keep core tight and maintain good posture throughout exercise
- ➡ Keep back flat and head in neutral position
- ➡ Avoid using body for momentum

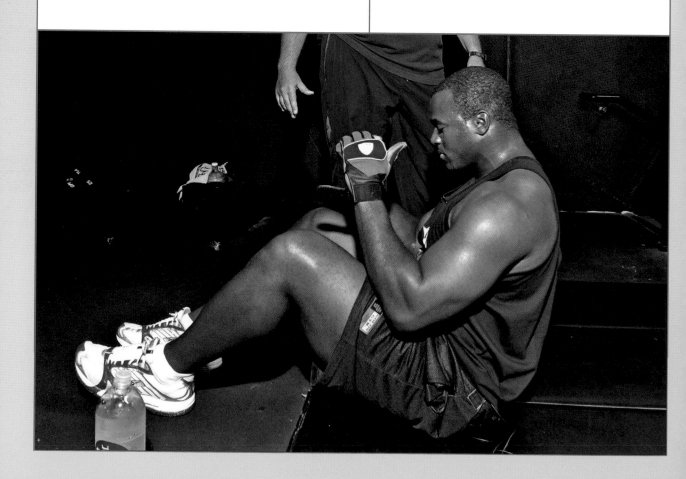

5 V CRUNCH

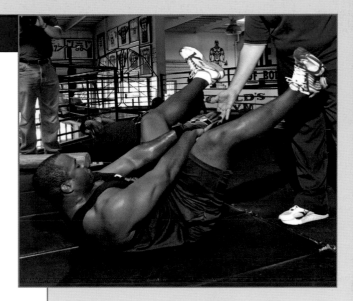

Hicks: With the legs being spread, it really helps with flexibility in his adductors and abductors.

• Lie with back on ground and legs pointing toward ceiling and spread apart

• Keeping arms straight, crunch up and forward between legs

• Lower with control; repeat for specified reps

COACHING POINTS

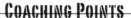

➡ Spread legs as far as possible, but remain comfortable

➡ Avoid letting legs drop too far forward

➡ Keep back flat and head in neutral position

➡ Avoid using body for momentum

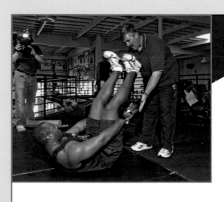

6 OUTSIDE THIGH REACH

Hicks: This gives him a little bit more shoulder flexion, because he has to bring his shoulders forward and then reach.

• Lie with back on ground and legs straight up toward ceiling

• Keeping arms straight, crunch up and forward while reaching arms around outside of thighs

• Lower with control; repeat for specified reps

COACHING POINTS

➡ Reach arms as far as possible outside of thighs

➡ Keep core tight and maintain good posture throughout exercise

➡ Keep back flat and head in neutral position

➡ Avoid using body for momentum

BUTTERFLY SIT-UP

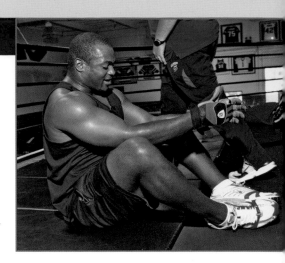

Hicks: This helps tremendously [by increasing] hip and lower abs strength.

- Assume sit-up position with knees wide and soles of feet touching each other

- Without rocking, perform sit-up

- Lower slowly until shoulder blades reach floor

- Repeat for specified reps

COACHING POINTS

➤ Keep core tight and maintain good posture throughout exercise

➤ Keep back flat and head in neutral position

➤ Avoid using body for momentum

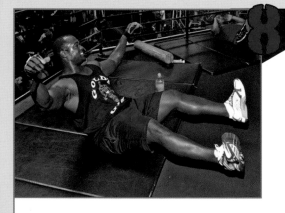

SPREAD EAGLE STABILITY HOLD

Hicks: This works stability in the low back and hips.

- Sitting on butt, assume spread eagle position with heels just off ground

- Hold position for specified duration

COACHING POINTS

➤ Keep lumbar spine [lower back] in straight line

➤ Keep core tight and maintain good posture throughout exercise

➤ Keep back flat and head in neutral position

➤ Avoid moving arms and body to maintain balance

9 OVERHEAD REACH STABILITY HOLD

Hicks: This really works shoulder stabilization and flexibility.

- Sitting on butt, bring knees to chest and extend arms straight overhead

- Hold position for specified duration

COACHING POINTS

➡ Make sure biceps are by ears and thumbs are locked overhead

➡ Keep core tight and maintain good posture throughout exercise

➡ Keep back flat and head in neutral position

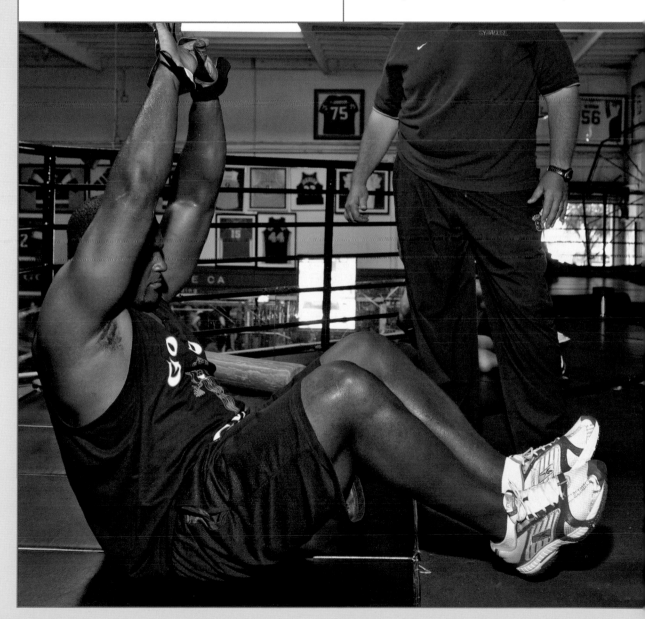

ALTERNATE DUMBBELL BENCH SEQUENCE

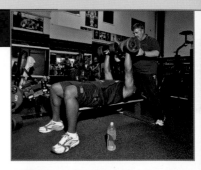

Hicks: When he's at the top, it's mainly chest and tricep. When the arm's at the bottom, it's chest and shoulders.

- Lie with back on bench, holding dumbbells in front of chest with palms slightly facing in

- Keeping left arm straight, lower right dumbbell to chest level, then drive it back to start position

- Keeping right arm straight, lower left dumbbell to chest level, then drive it back to start position

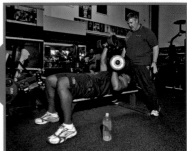

- Repeat for specified reps

- Lower both dumbbells within an inch from chest and perform same alternating sequence while holding opposite dumbbell at low position

- Immediately perform standard presses with both dumbbells for specified reps

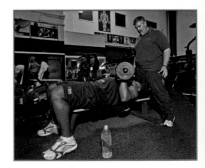

COACHING POINTS

- ➡ Go through full range of motion
- ➡ Hold dumbbell you aren't using at midline of chest
- ➡ Keep back flat and head in neutral position
- ➡ Avoid using body for momentum

DUMBBELL INCLINE

Hicks: This hits a different part of the chest, which will lead us into hitting his shoulders.

- Assume position on incline bench with dumbbells at shoulders

- Without arching back, drive dumbbells toward ceiling until arms are fully extended

- Lower dumbbells with control to start position; repeat for specified reps

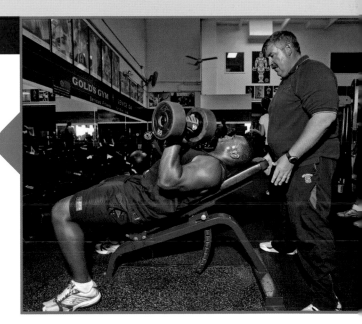

COACHING POINTS

- ➤ Go through full range of motion
- ➤ Use weight that makes movement difficult, not impossible
- ➤ Keep movement within framework of body
- ➤ Keep back flat and head in neutral position
- ➤ Avoid using body for momentum

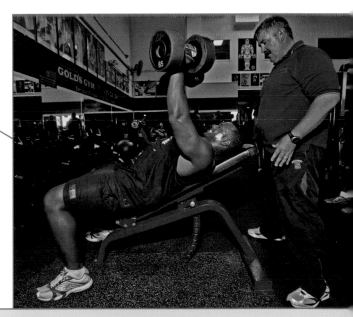

PLYO PUSH-UP SERIES

Hicks: The reason we do three different movements—the clap your hand, then the chest slap or the alternate side-to-side—is to give you some stability in the shoulder joint and to give you structure within a workout, where you get in an unnatural position. It's basically plyometrics for the upper body.

PLYO PUSH-UP WITH CLAP

- Assume push-up position and lower body until chest almost touches ground

- Explosively drive body up by fully extending arms

- Clap hands together in front of chest

- Land with hands shoulder-width apart; immediately perform next rep

- Perform continuously for specified reps

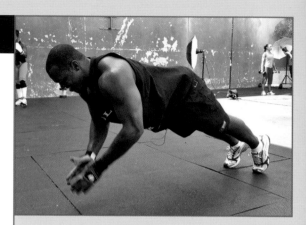

PLYO PUSH-UP WITH CHEST SLAP

- Assume push-up position and lower body until chest almost touches ground

- Explosively drive body up by fully extending arms

- Slap both hands to chest

- Land with hands shoulder-width apart; immediately perform next rep

- Perform continuously for specified reps

3 PLYO PUSH-UP SIDE-TO-SIDE WITH CLAP

- Assume push-up position and lower body until chest almost touches ground

- Explosively drive body up and left by fully extending arms

- Clap hands together in front of chest

- Land left of starting position with hands at shoulder width

- Immediately perform next rep up and back to right

- Perform continuously for specified reps

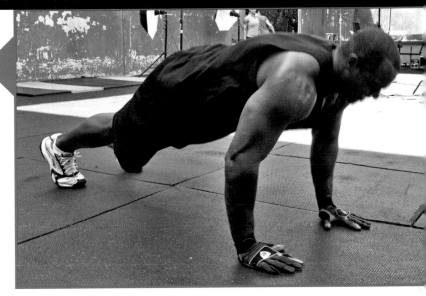

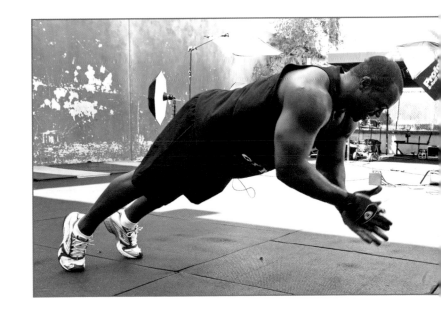

COACHING POINTS

➡ Keep core tight and maintain good posture throughout exercise

➡ Keep back flat and head in neutral position

➡ Push up off ground as explosively as possible

4 DUMBBELL CLEAN, RIP, AND PRESS

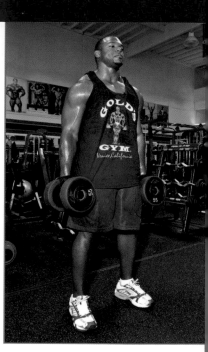

Hicks: It's a total body movement, and we do it on the shoulder day because of the press aspect. It's a great exercise, because to be able to perform it, your whole body has to fire properly.

• Assume athletic stance holding dumbbells at sides

• Explosively extend hips, knees, and ankles while simultaneously shrugging

• Drive elbows toward ceiling, bringing dumbbells to shoulder level

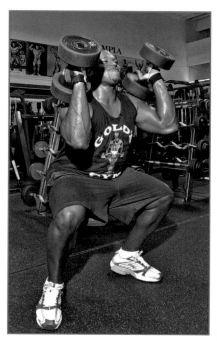

• Catch dumbbells at shoulders in squat position

• Explosively extend hips, knees, and ankles while driving dumbbells overhead

• Finish in athletic stance with arms fully extended overhead

• Return to start position with control; repeat for specified reps

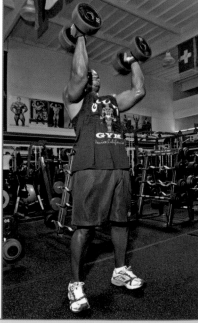

COACHING POINTS

➤ Land with feet flat on ground
➤ Keep hips underneath body throughout exercise
➤ Maintain balance throughout exercise

DUMBBELL SHOULDER CIRCUIT

Hicks: We're just trying to train all three heads of the deltoid—basically building some strength around the shoulder joint to keep him healthy. It's more of an injury prevention circuit than a power output movement.

DUMBBELL LATERAL RAISES
For the medial delt

- Assume athletic stance with dumbbells at sides

- Without rocking or changing body position, raise dumbbells out to side until arms are parallel to ground

- Lower dumbbells with control; repeat for specified reps

- Perform in circuit with front and rear delt raises

COACHING POINTS

- ► Keep elbows slightly higher than wrists
- ► Avoid turning movement into a fly
- ► Keep core tight and maintain good posture throughout exercise
- ► Keep back flat and head in neutral position

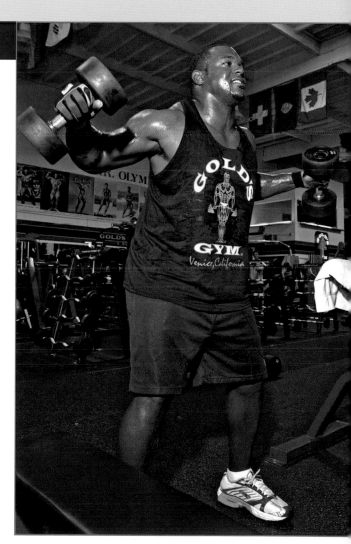

DUMBBELL FRONT RAISES
For the anterior delt

- Assume athletic stance with dumbbells at sides

- Without rocking or changing body position, raise dumbbells in front until arms are parallel to ground

- Lower dumbbells with control; repeat for specified reps

- Perform in circuit with lateral and rear delt raises

COACHING POINTS

- ➡ Keep elbows slightly higher than wrists
- ➡ Keep core tight and maintain good posture throughout exercise
- ➡ Keep back flat and head in neutral position
- ➡ Avoid using body for momentum

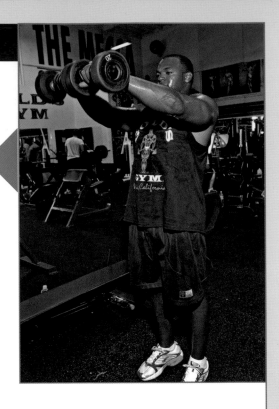

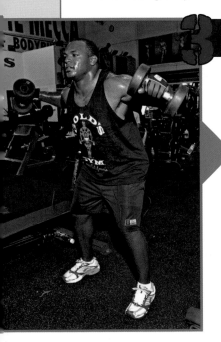

DUMBBELL REAR DELT RAISES WITH PUNCH
For the posterior delt

- Assume athletic stance and bend forward until chest is almost parallel to ground

- Without rocking or changing body position, bring dumbbells out to sides until they are parallel to ground

- Keeping arms out to sides, perform punch by pushing each dumbbell away from body

- Lower dumbbells with control; repeat for specified reps

- Perform in circuit with lateral and front raises

COACHING POINTS

- ➡ Keep elbows slightly higher than wrists   ➡ Keep core tight and maintain good posture throughout exercise
- ➡ Keep back flat and head in neutral position   ➡ Avoid using body for momentum

4 MACHINE HANG SHRUGS
For overall power output through the triple extension

- In athletic stance, grasp handles of shrug machine [or barbell if machine is unavailable]

- Explosively extend hips, knees and ankles while shrugging straight arms

- Return to start position; repeat for specified reps

COACHING POINTS

➡ Avoid bringing neck down instead of shoulders up
➡ Avoid rolling shoulders forward
➡ Maintain balance throughout exercise
➡ Bring shoulders to ears

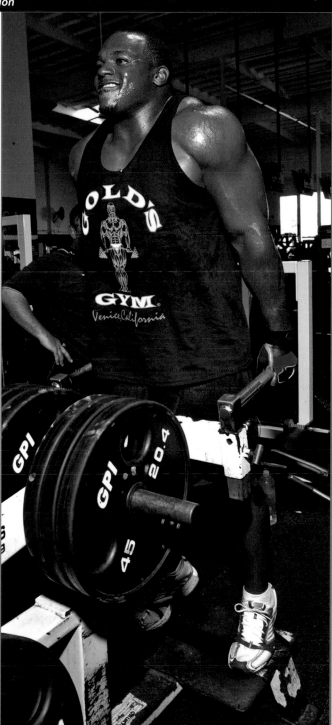

TRICEP CIRCUIT

Hicks: Basically, what we're trying to do is work the long, middle, and inner head of the tricep. We like to do the tricep circuit to pre-fatigue his triceps before we do an athletic-related tricep movement using a med ball.

TRICEP PUSHDOWN

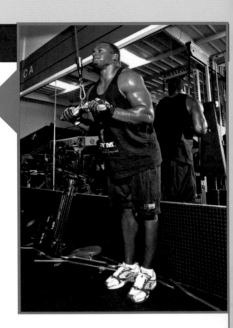

- In athletic stance facing cable machine, hold pushdown attachment in front of sternum

- Keeping elbows tight to ribs, drive handle down until arms are fully extended

- Return arms to start position with control; repeat for specified reps

- Perform in circuit with underhand and overhead extensions

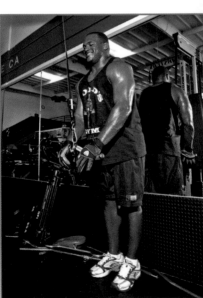

COACHING POINTS

- ➤ Perform with overhand grip slightly narrower than shoulder width
- ➤ Keep elbows pinned tightly to sides during movement
- ➤ Keep head up and back flat
- ➤ Avoid using body for momentum

UNDERHAND TRICEP EXTENSION

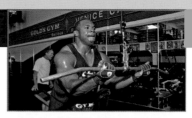

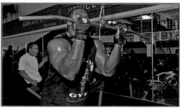

- In athletic stance a few feet from cable machine, hold lat pulldown bar with underhand grip

- Keeping elbows out in front of body, drive bar straight down and away from body until arms are fully extended

- Return arms to start position with control; repeat for specified reps

- Perform in circuit with pushdowns and overhead extensions

COACHING POINTS

➤ Keep head up and back flat
➤ Avoid using body for momentum
➤ Keeps abs tight, shoulders back, and chest up throughout exercise
➤ Avoid letting elbows flare out to sides

OVERHEAD TRICEP EXTENSION

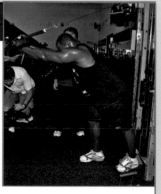

- In split stance with back to cable machine, hold rope attachment overhead

- Keeping forward body lean, fully extend arms

- Return arms to start position with control; repeat for specified reps

- Perform in circuit with pushdowns and underhand extensions

COACHING POINTS

➤ Perform entire exercise with control
➤ Keep head up and back flat
➤ Avoid using body for momentum
➤ Avoid letting elbows splay out to sides

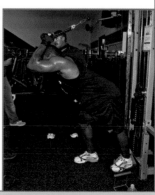

4 SINGLE-ARM PHYSIOBALL PUSH-UP

• Assume push-up position with one hand on small physioball or large med ball

• Perform push-ups for specified reps; repeat set with opposite hand on ball

COACHING POINTS

➡ Keep back flat and hips underneath body
➡ Keep hand flat on ball and on ground
➡ Maintain balance throughout exercise

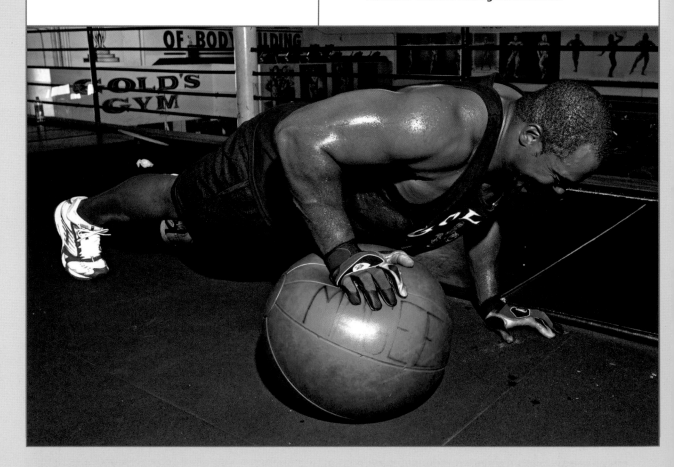

DWIGHT FREENEY'S TRAINING GUIDE

CORE WARM-UP

	SETS/REPS	REST IN SECONDS	NOTES
Toe Touches	1x20	35-45	
Single-Leg Toe Touches	1x20 each leg	35-45	
Single-Leg Reach Through	1x20 each leg	35-45	
Full Sit-Up	1x10	35-45	
V Crunch	1x20	35-45	
Outside Thigh Reach	1x20	35-45	
Butterfly Sit-Up	1x10	35-45	
Spread Eagle Stability Hold	1x10 seconds	35-45	
Overhead Reach Stability Hold	1x10 seconds	35-45	

2-minute recovery

STRENGTH

	SETS/REPS	REST IN SECONDS	NOTES
Alternate Dumbbell Bench Sequence	1x6+6+6; 1x5+5+5 1x4+4+4	35-45	
Dumbbell Incline	1x10, 1x8, 1x6	35-45	

2-minute recovery

PLYO PUSH-UP SERIES

	SETS/REPS	REST IN SECONDS	NOTES
Plyo Push-Up With Clap	1x8	35-45	
Plyo Push-Up With Chest Slap	1x8	35-45	
Plyo Push-Up Side to Side With Clap	1x8 (4 each way)	35-45	
Dumbbell Clean, Rip, and Press	3x6	35-45	

2-minute recovery

DUMBBELL SHOULDER CIRCUIT

	SETS/REPS	REST IN SECONDS	NOTES
Dumbbell Lateral Raises	2x8	0	Perform as part of circuit
Dumbbell Front Raises	2x8	0	Perform as part of circuit
Dumbbell Rear Delt Raises With Punch	2x8	0	Perform as part of circuit
Machine Hang Shrugs	3x20-25	35-45	

2-minute recovery

TRICEP CIRCUIT

	SETS/REPS	REST IN SECONDS	NOTES
Tricep Pushdown	3x8-10	0	2x8 each arm
Underhand Tricep Extension	3x8-10	0	2x8 each arm
Overhead Tricep Extension	3x8-10	0	2x8 each arm
Single-Arm Physioball Push-Up	2x8 each arm	35-45	

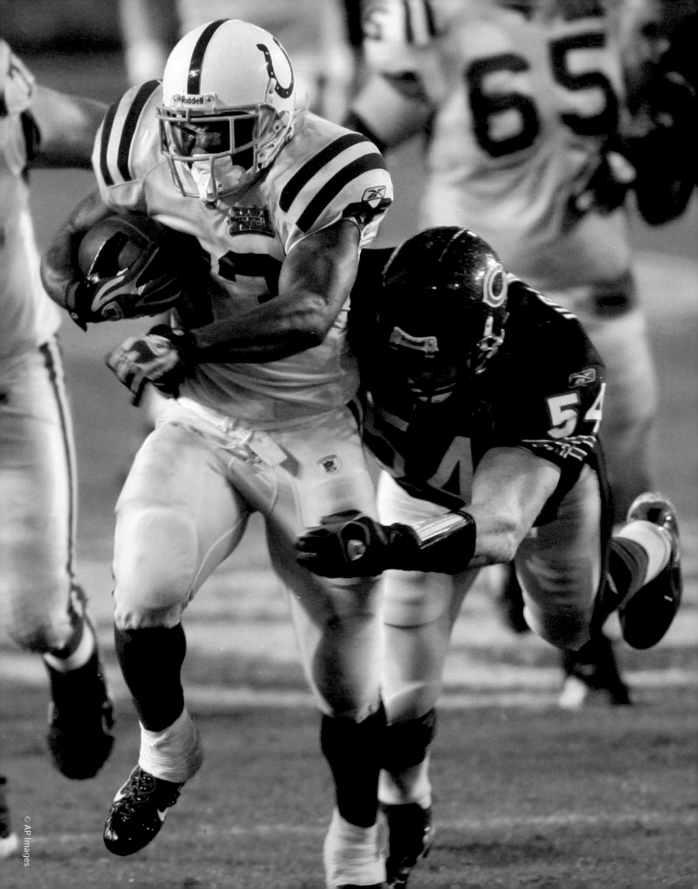

CHAPTER 10

BRIAN URLACHER

EDITOR'S NOTE

Butkus. Singletary. Following in the footsteps of two Monsters of the Midway, legends known simply by their surnames and slobber-knocker hits, is no easy chore. But since his introduction into the Windy City in 1998, Brian Urlacher has clawed his way into the discussion as one of the best linebackers ever to don the Bears' emblematic wishbone "C."

Carrying the torch ignited by Butkus and kept burning with fury by Singletary requires discipline, commitment, and revolutionary training. Instead of resting on his impressive workout regimen and unparalleled early NFL laurels, Urlacher, a former University of New Mexico standout, added fuel to his off-season training fire by working out with legendary coach Chip Smith. The results? An outstanding 2005 season, filled with lighting up the opposition and highlighted by a Defensive Player of the Year Award.

Before the 2004 season, Urlacher's agent had contacted nationally renowned speed and strength specialist Chip Smith about improving the linebacker's game-day endurance. Although

BRIAN URLACHER DIVE-TACKLES THE COLTS' DOMINIC RHODES DURING SUPER BOWL XLI IN 2007. HIGH-ALTITUDE WORKOUTS HAVE IMPROVED URLACHER'S ENDURANCE.

he had been tabbed to four straight Pro Bowls to start his stellar career, the Bears' leader wanted to gain an additional competitive edge.

After much deliberation about training Urlacher outside his Atlanta complex, Smith went to work developing an unheard-of high-altitude training program. Not only did the speed sensei have to consider the side effects of training thousands of feet above sea level, he also had to create a regimen that would ensure Urlacher's high-end stamina would last all four quarters. Furthermore, the program needed to maintain Urlacher's off-season strength gains and meet his caloric and protein dietary requirements.

All complex demands to meet, but when an elite athlete desires to improve every facet of his game, unprecedented evolutionary thinking is required. The two conditioning mavericks packed up shop and headed west, down a lightly traveled road, for a training adventure full of exciting prospects. What transpired over the course of four weeks high in the mountains of Lake Tahoe was a revolutionary method of football training validated by results that exceeded performance expectations.

Smith's story, relaying his first-hand account of high-altitude training with Urlacher and the complementary weight room work he used to maintain Urlacher's muscle strength and increase his muscle endurance, ran in the March 2005 issue of *STACK*.

Here, you'll read Smith's explanation of the training and learn how Urlacher is still adding to his Hall of Fame resume, thanks in large part to his emphasis on off-field preparation, which has continued since he joined Smith. You'll also see why Urlacher has extinguished all debates surrounding his status as one of the best linebackers in the game.

INTO THIN AIR

Why High Altitude Training?

Air in higher altitudes has less oxygen. When there isn't much oxygen in the air, hypoxia, which is oxygen deprivation in muscle tissue, occurs, causing muscles to fatigue quicker.

The effects are only temporary, because the body produces erythropoietin [EPO]. EPO causes the body to produce additional red blood cells, which carry oxygen-rich blood to muscles for additional energy. When Urlacher returns to normal sea level, his extra red blood cells can transport more oxygen than normal, which delays muscle fatigue—exactly what he wants in the fourth quarter for longer, harder play and faster recovery.

The Design Challenge

Urlacher wanted me to design a program to help improve his fourth-quarter endurance. I've always trained Urlacher position-specific by having him work on scraping and filing, pursuit, first-step explosion, pass drops, change-of-direction, and any other drills to benefit his position.

After reviewing film of four games, I had to locate the reasons why Urlacher was tiring so much in the third and fourth quarters. What stuck out the most from the film was how much he ran on each play. I circled and put a stopwatch on the end of each play. Urlacher ran to the ball every play. No matter if it was a run or pass, he was in the circle within three seconds of every play. The amount of his sprinting was substantial.

After watching game cuts for days, I designed a game- and movement-specific program, which included aerobic work for duration and anaerobic for short explosive bursts. To address resistance in his training—to mimic obstacles on the field—I implemented a quick-release handle, which gave Urlacher resistance without impeding his movement. For example, when he blitzed or played the run, he faced resistance equivalent to taking on a center or guard, which endured for four or five steps. Once he moved up field three yards, I released the resistance, at which point he turned and sprinted 15 yards.

Weight Work

The next consideration for Urlacher's summer program was his weight work. I wanted to increase his aerobic endurance as well as his muscle endurance while maintaining the strength gains he made during his off-season workouts in Chicago.

So, to keep the main goal of his weight program in sight, which was to increase muscle endurance, I had to figure out at what intensity he could train without overdoing it. To keep it simple, I broke Urlacher's workouts into a

push-pull regimen and constantly changed the reps, sets, and exercises. I kept Urlacher's rest time at 25 seconds [huddle time] between each set and one minute between each exercise. This type of high-volume training helped achieve muscle endurance and fat burning, which is what Urlacher wanted.

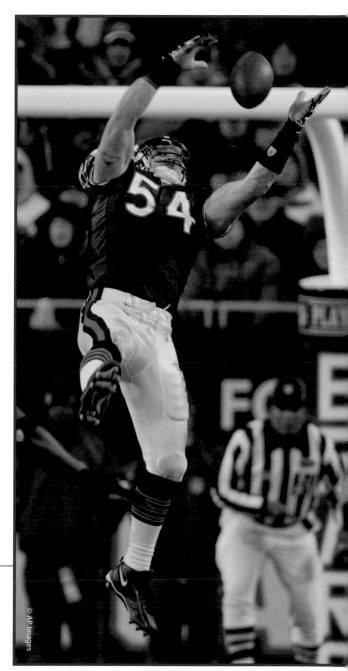

© AP Images

Diet

The last challenge to contend with was Urlacher's diet. I wanted to ensure that training at high altitude didn't result in loss of lean muscle, so I based Urlacher's dietary needs on a couple of factors. First were his caloric needs, and second his protein needs. After some complicated testing, I determined Urlacher needed roughly 3,840 calories per day during training. Due to his activity level, I added another 2,000 calories per day to increase the intake to 5,800 calories per day.

Urlacher also needed to get enough protein to offset the effects of high-volume training and explosive running. So, I simply based his protein needs on one gram of protein per pound of body weight, which meant he needed 256 grams per day. However, requiring that much protein intake can cause a problem. A body can assimilate 30 grams per meal; so, I had to figure out how Urlacher could get all 256 protein grams. To solve the problem, I used ready-to-drink protein shakes. About every three hours, Urlacher drank a shake or ate a meal.

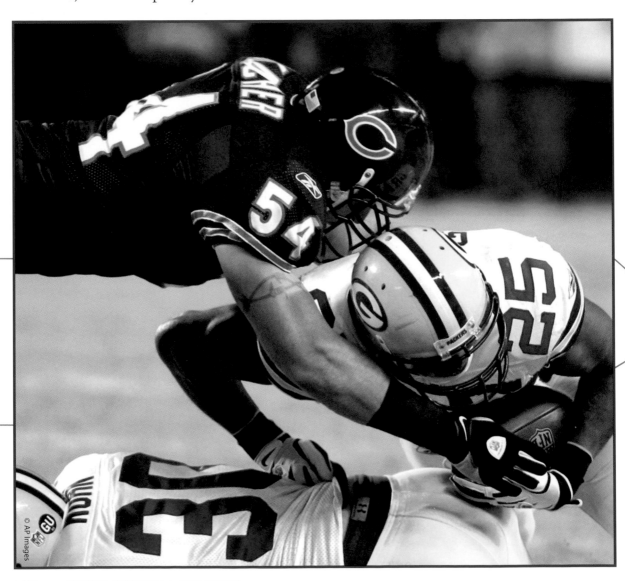

© AP Images

Final Results

Slow-twitch muscle fibers contract slowly, but they can sustain contractions for long periods of time without fatiguing; they get most energy from burning fat. Pure fast-twitch fibers contract rapidly, but they fatigue quickly. Their energy comes mostly from burning glycogen. Urlacher definitely has more fast-twitch fibers than slow-twitch ones.

However, as with the slow-twitch fiber, fast-twitch fibers can also burn fat. So high-volume training can help change pure fast-twitch fibers into fast-twitch oxidative fibers that burn fat at a faster rate. With the combination of explosive running and weight work, Urlacher's body literally became a fat-burning machine over the course of four weeks. Below are pre-workout measurements taken on June 26, 2004, and then the final results after four weeks on July 26, 2004:

June 26, 2004

Body weight: 256 pounds
Bodypod measurement for body composition: 6.9% body fat
Exercising heart rate:
173 beats per minute
Three-minute recovery:
118 beats per minute
315-pound max reps for Bench Press:
8 reps

July 26, 2004

Body weight: 255.3 pounds
Bodypod measurement for body composition: 4.9% body fat
Exercising heart rate:
172 beats per minute
Three-minute recovery:
80 beats per minute
315-pound max reps on Bench Press:
12 reps

Basically, Urlacher lowered his body fat by two percent, which is roughly about 5.10 pounds of total fat loss. Also, he increased his lung capacity by two percent, which allows for better stamina on the field, and improved four reps on his 315-pound bench-press max. These improvements confirmed the results we anticipated from the outset.

EXERCISES

TURN AND RUN

Setup: Place mini discs on ground to resemble offensive line

- Attach resistance cord around waist

- Assume position-specific athletic stance

- On verbal command, turn right and run down the line as if pursuing a play on the outside

- Repeat movement to left

Sets/Rest: 2 x each direction; 45-second rest between sets

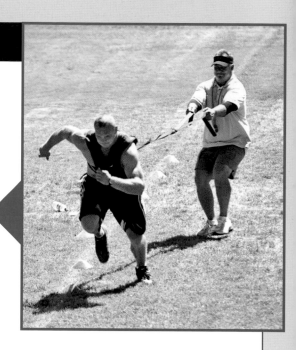

FORWARD BURST

Setup: Place mini discs on ground to resemble offensive line

- Attach resistance cord around waist

- Assume position-specific athletic stance

- On verbal command, burst forward and fill designated gap

- Vary forward bust-gap movements

Sets/Rest: 2 x each gap; 45-second rest between sets

3 BACKPEDAL

- Assume position-specific athletic stance

- On verbal command, backpedal 15 yards

Sets/Rest: 2; 45-second rest

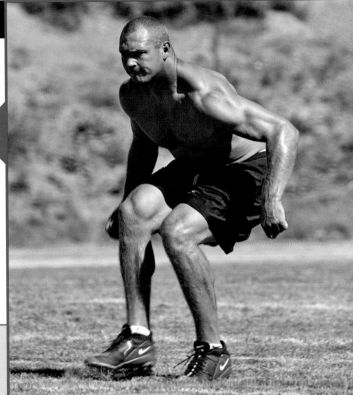

4 BACKPEDAL BREAK

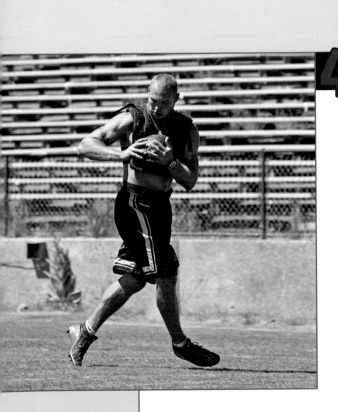

- Assume position-specific athletic stance

- On verbal command, backpedal 10 yards; on visual command, break forward at 45-degree angle left or right

- Catch ball

Adaptation: Use 45-degree angle forward/backward breaks and flat breaks

Sets/Rest: 2 x each direction; 45-second rest

CHEST, BACK, AND BICEPS

1 BENCH PRESS

- Lie down on bench and grip bar slightly wider than shoulder width

- Lower bar until it touches slightly below pectorals at base of sternum

- Drive bar straight up off chest until arms are fully extended

- Repeat for specified reps

COACHING POINTS

- Avoid bouncing bar off chest
- Keep back and butt on bench
- Inhale on way down; exhale while exploding bar up

2 SEATED ROW

- Sit at seated row machine with arms extended in front

- Place hands on grips shoulder-width apart with palms facing each other or pointed toward ground

- Pull arms back, driving elbows back past body

- Control weight back to start position

- Repeat for specified reps

COACHING POINTS

- Avoid rocking back to gain momentum

3 INCLINE PRESS

- Lie down on incline bench and grip bar slightly wider than shoulder width

- Lower bar until it touches top half of pectoral

- Drive bar straight up off chest until arms are fully extended

- Repeat for specified reps

COACHING POINTS

- Avoid bouncing bar off chest
- Keep body on bench entire time
- Inhale on way down; exhale while exploding bar up

4 ONE-ARM ROW

- Place left foot on ground and right knee on bench

- Lean forward until back is parallel to ground; place right hand on bench with arm straight and elbow locked

- Hold dumbbell in left hand with palm facing body

- Drive elbow toward ceiling to bring dumbbell to chest

- Control weight back to start position

- Repeat for specified reps

COACHING POINTS

- ➤ Avoid jerking dumbbell back during movement
- ➤ Keep knee on bench entire time
- ➤ Use slow, controlled movements
- ➤ Pull elbow back as far as possible

5 DIPS

- Start with arms near sides with elbows and shoulders locked

- Lower body until shoulders are only inches above hands

- Push body back up to start position

- Repeat for specified reps

COACHING POINTS

- ➤ Focus on full range of motion
- ➤ Avoid kicking feet
- ➤ Do not use lower body for momentum

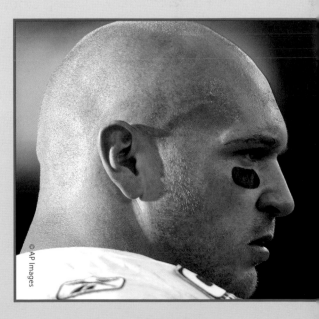

© AP Images

6 LAT PULLDOWN

- Sit with slight backward lean

- Grip bar with slightly wider than shoulder-width grip and palms facing away from body

- Use elbows and back to pull down until bar passes chin

- Control bar back to start position

- Repeat for specified reps

COACHING POINTS

- Use slow, controlled movements while lowering bar
- Avoid rocking back to gain momentum
- Focus on full range of motion
- Do not sit back further than 45-degree angle

7 STRAIGHT BAR CURL

- Stand with bar at thigh level and use slightly wider than hip-width grip with palms facing away from body

- Lock upper arms in place and curl bar to chest

- Lower bar back to start position

- Repeat for specified reps

COACHING POINTS

Focus on using arms to lift bar
Do not sway or lean forward to gain momentum
Use full range of motion
Squeeze biceps while raising bar

8 SEATED DB CURLS

- Sit at end of bench with dumbbell in each hand

- Start with arms straight down and palms facing away from body

- Keep upper arms in place and curl dumbbells to shoulders

- Lower dumbbells back to start position

- Repeat for specified reps

COACHING POINTS

- Focus on using arms to lift dumbbells
- Do not rock back to gain momentum
- Use full range of motion
- Squeeze biceps while lifting dumbbells
- Use slow, controlled movements

9 CRUNCHES

- Lie on ground with feet flat on floor with slight bend in knees

- Place hands behind head

- Use abs to lift shoulders and upper back off ground

- Lower to start position

- Repeat for specified reps

COACHING POINTS

Isolate abs while lifting body
Squeeze abdominal muscles during entire set
Avoid using hands as catalyst to crunch
Keep feet flat on floor entire set

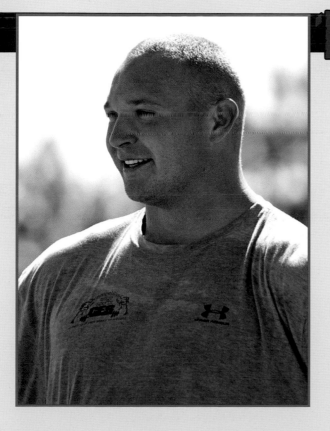

10 KNEE-UPS

- Hang from pull-up bar

- Use abs to lift knees to chest without swinging

- Lower knees to start position

- Repeat for specified reps

COACHING POINTS

➤ Use slow, controlled movements while raising and lowering legs
➤ Do not swing to gain momentum
➤ Concentrate on full range of motion

TRICEPS, SHOULDERS, AND LEGS

CLEANS

- Stand with barbell at thigh level

- Grip bar at hip width with palms facing toward body

- Bend knees and push hips back

- Explode up and extend at ankles, hips, and knees

- Shrug shoulders and pull bar straight up

- Begin to bend arms and continue to pull on bar while dropping hips

- Catch bar across shoulders and chest in squat position

- Drive up from squat until standing straight up

- Repeat for specified reps

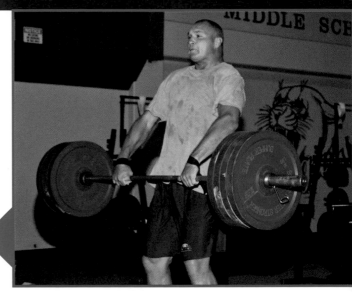

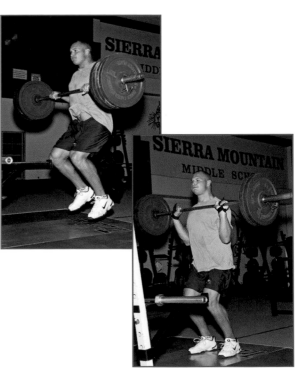

COACHING POINTS

- Keep bar over toes
- Engage hip flexors, quads, and lower back
- Keep shoulders up and back
- Get hips down and under bar in one smooth movement
- Drop under bar to catch it safely

2 SHRUGS

- Stand with bar at thigh level

- Grip bar at hip width with palms facing toward body

- Keeping arms straight, lift up on bar by shrugging shoulders toward ears

- Lower bar back to start position

- Repeat for specified reps

COACHING POINTS

Use trap muscles to shrug bar
Do not use arms to lift bar
Avoid rolling shoulders forward
   or backward

3 LEG EXTENSION

- Sit at extension machine with legs bent 90 degrees

- Straighten legs until fully extended

- Lower legs back to starting position

- Repeat for specified reps

COACHING POINTS

- ➤ Avoid swinging legs upward for momentum
- ➤ Resist machine slowly on way down

4 SQUATS

- Position underneath bar in squat rack so bar sits on traps, slightly below base of neck

- Set feet slightly wider than shoulder-width apart and toes slightly pointed out

- Looking straight ahead, unrack bar and squat until thighs are parallel to ground

- Pushing through heels, drive weight up to start position

- Repeat for specified reps

COACHING POINTS

- ➤ Focus eyes straight ahead
- ➤ Keep back flat
- ➤ Avoid collapsing knees on way down
- ➤ Do not lean forward

5 SEATED MILITARY PRESS

- Sit on bench with bar at chest level

- Use a slightly wider than shoulder-width grip with palms facing away from body

- Push bar straight overhead until arms are fully extended

- Lower bar back down to chest

- Repeat for specified reps

COACHING POINTS

- ➤ Keep core tight and avoid leaning forward or back
- ➤ Use full range of motion

6 FRONT RAISES

- Stand with arms straight down and palms facing body with dumbbells in each hand

- Raise arms in front of body until parallel to ground

- Lower dumbbells to start position

- Repeat for specified reps

COACHING POINTS

- ➤ Do not go past point of pain
- ➤ Do not sway or use lower body for momentum
- ➤ Hold dumbbells in raised position for two seconds

7 UPRIGHT ROW

- Stand with bar or curl bar at thigh level

- Place hands on bar six to eight inches apart with palms facing body

- Leading with elbows, pull bar up toward chin

- Lower bar to start position

- Repeat for specified reps

COACHING POINTS

- ➤ Avoid rocking body back and forth
- ➤ Use full range of motion

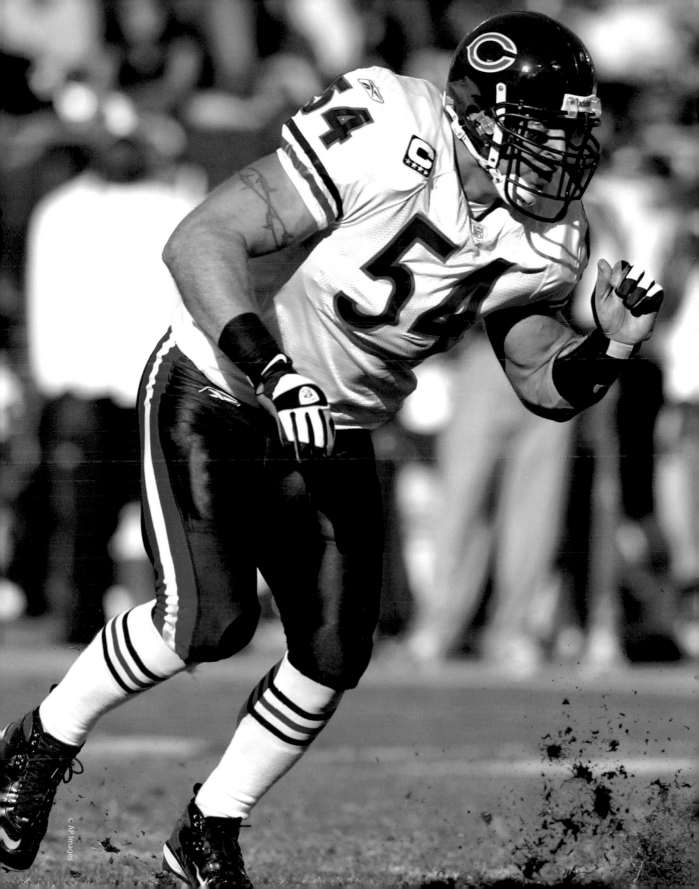

8 SIDE LATERAL RAISE

- Stand with arms straight down and facing each other with dumbbells in each hand

- Keeping arms straight, raise them out to sides until parallel to ground

- Lower dumbbells to start position

- Repeat for specified reps

COACHING POINTS

➡ Keep arms as straight as possible

➡ Use slow, controlled movements

9 TRICEP EXTENSION

- Lie on back on bench, gripping bar or curl bar with hands no more than six to eight inches apart and arms fully extended above chest

- Lower bar toward head bending at elbows only

- Lower bar until it nearly touches head between eyes and top of forehead

- Use triceps to drive bar back to start position

- Repeat for specified reps

COACHING POINTS

➡ Focus on using triceps and arms ➡ Keep arms locked at shoulders

10 CLOSE-GRIP BENCH PRESS

- Lie on back on bench

- Place hands on bar eight to 12 inches apart, so hands are inside shoulder width

- Lower bar until it touches base of sternum

- Keep arms tight and drive bar straight up until arms are fully extended

- Repeat for specified reps

COACHING POINTS

➡ Do not bounce bar off chest

➡ Focus on full range of motion

➡ Keep back and butt on bench entire time

BRIAN URLACHER'S TRAINING GUIDE

CHEST, BACK, AND BICEPS

Treat each pairing of exercises in both workouts as a superset. To superset exercises, complete a set of one exercise, rest 25 seconds, and immediately perform a set of the second exercise. For example, complete 8 reps of Incline Press, rest, and then complete 8 reps of One-Arm Row.

	SETS/REPS
Bench Press	4 x 3
Seated Row	4 x 8
Incline Press	4 x 8
One-Arm Row	4 x 8
Dips	3 x as many as possible
Lat Pulldown	3 x 12
Straight Bar Curl	1 x 10, 1 x 8, 3 x 6
Seated DB Curls	3 x 8
Crunches	3 x 30
Knee-Ups	3 x 30

TRICEPS, SHOULDERS, AND LEGS

Treat each pairing of exercises in both workouts as a superset. To superset exercises, complete a set of one exercise, rest 25, and immediately perform a set of the second exercise. For example, complete 12 reps of Leg Extensions, rest, and then complete 6 reps of Squats.

	SETS/REPS
Cleans	1 x 10, 1 x 8, 3 x 6
Shrugs	4 x 8
Leg Extension	3 x 12
Squats	4 x 6
Seated Military Press	4 x 10
Front Raises	4 x 8
Upright Row	4 x 8
Side Lateral Raise	4 x 8
Tricep Extension	1 x 10, 1 x 8, 1 x 6, 1 x 4
Close-Grip Bench Press	1 x 10, 1 x 8, 1 x 6, 1 x 4

RECOMMENDED RESOURCES

STACK

For the Athlete, By the Athlete

Originally founded as a magazine, STACK has developed into a fully diversified multimedia company providing information and advice on athletic training, nutrition, and sports skills from top professional and collegiate athletes and coaches on the following major brand platforms:

STACK Media is one of the top sports properties on the Internet, with an average of four million unique visitors and 100 million page views per month. Combining its editorial content with product and service offerings from several partner sites in a distributed media network, STACK Media has become the acknowledged leader in reaching its audience of active sports participants online.

STACK.com, the digital home for all STACK content and web-based tools, is one of the Internet's fastest growing sites, delivering information exclusively for the active sports community.

STACK TV, an online video platform with eight channels of unique, originally produced videos, delivers the largest library of sports performance video content on the web.

STACK Magazine, requested by more than 9,000 high school athletic directors, has a circulation of 800,000 and a readership of more than five million high school athletes.

MySTACK, a social network and recruiting site that allows athletes to create profiles with their personal information and stats, upload highlight films and photos, and send their profiles to college coaches to take control of the recruiting process.

Eastbay [Eastbay.com]

The leading supplier of athletic footwear, apparel, and training gear, Eastbay.com and its direct mail catalog are essential resources for athletes interested in the top brands, including Nike, Reebok, adidas, and others. As marketing partners, STACK and Eastbay share the goal of helping high school and college athletes meet all of their performance needs. Through Eastbay Training Centers, presented by STACK on Eastbay.com, the retailer offers the latest and greatest in sport performance content as well as its traditional product lines.

beRecruited.com

Founded in 2000 by a former collegiate athlete, beRecruited.com provides a platform for high school student-athletes to connect and interact with college coaches across the nation. More than 200,000 registered student-athletes use beRecruited.com to build online profiles and evaluate opportunities to take their game to the next level. STACK creates content to inform high school athletes of the recruiting process, while beRecruited offers an environment in which athletes can apply their skills and knowledge to achieve their recruiting goals.

Varsity Networks, Inc. [varsitynetworks.com]
Varsity Networks helps more than 9,000 high schools across the country manage, motivate, and stay connected with their teams. Users are able to post commentary, video, photos, and team stats to the site. The company also distributes content to local and national media outlets to feature on-air or on their websites. Varsity Network's services have value for all members of the high school sports community, including athletic directors, coaches, players, parents, and fans.

iHigh.com
iHigh.com, Inc. offers free services to high schools and student-athletes throughout the United States, allowing them to create and maintain their own branded websites. Through iHigh.com, teams and news organizations are able to post live broadcasts, stories, photos, and videos to their customized team pages. Student-athletes can also set up individual profiles through the social network myihigh.com. The iHigh site features the first national network of member schools in one comprehensive online destination.

RECRUITING RESOURCES

National Collegiate Athletic Association [ncaa.org]
The NCAA's official website houses its Eligibility Center, which provides information and resources for prospective collegiate student-athletes. The NCAA Eligibility Center offers a guide for college-bound student-athletes, lists of approved high school academic requirements, and registration forms. Also available at ncaa.org is information on legislation and governance, statistics and records for all NCAA sports, and a comprehensive library of NCAA publications and journals.

NUTRITION RESOURCES

Gatorade Sports Science Institute [GSSI] [gssiweb.com]
GSSI is a research facility dedicated to sharing the latest information about exercise science and sports nutrition. In an effort to expand education about enhancing athletic performance, the Institute provides services and tools for athletes and sports health professionals and develops state-of-the-art technology used by the nation's principal scientists who are committed to furthering sports nutrition research.

Other Resources

Chip Smith
Competitive Edge Sports, Duluth, Georgia [competitiveedgesports.com]
*Football Training Like the Pros: Get Bigger, Stronger, and Faster Following the
    Programs of Today's Top Players.* Chip Smith, New York: McGraw-Hill [1998]

Danny Arnold
Plex, Stafford, Texas [plex.cc]
The Danny Arnold Show. Airs Saturdays at 8:00 a.m., Houston, Texas, 1560
    AM

Terrell Owens
*T.O.'s Finding Fitness: Making the Mind, Body, and Spirit Connection For Total
    Health.* Terrell Owens, B. Primm & C. Parker, New York: Simon & Schuster
    [2008]
Catch This!: Going Deep With The NFL's Sharpest Weapon. Terrell Owens & S.
    Singular, New York: Simon & Schuster [2004]
T.O. Terrell Owens & J. Rosenhaus, New York: Simon & Schuster [2006]
Little T Learns To Share. Terrell Owens, C. Parker & T. Harris, Dallas, Texas:
    BenBella Books [2006]
Bodylastics: The Terrell Owens Super Strong Man Edition [$100, tobands.
    com].
Making Of Champions Football Camp DVD. [$7, terrellowens.com]

Todd Durkin
Fitness Quest 10, San Diego, California [fitnessquest10.com]
TD Sports Performance DVD Series. L. Magill, T. Durkin, & B. Eveland, San Diego,
    Calif.: Time Zone Multimedia [2006]. [$245, fitnessquest10.com]
Speed Improvement Techniques for Young Athletes L. Magill, T. Durkin & B.
    Eveland, San Diego, Calif.: Time Zone Multimedia [2004].
Speed Improvement Techniques for Advanced Athletes L. Magill, T. Durkin, & B.
    Eveland, San Diego, Calif.: Time Zone Multimedia [2004].
Train the High School Athlete. V. Gabrielle & T. Durkin

Tom Shaw [coachtomshaw.com]
SPARQ Football Training DVD: $10
SPARQ Shaw 360 resistance trainer: $100
SPARQ Shaw 360 Belts: $10
SPARQ Shaw 360 Big Man's Belt: $5

Will Bartholomew [D1sportstraining.com]
D1 Sports Training: Nashville; Memphis; Huntsville; Little Rock; Greenville,
    South Carolina; Chattanooga; Knoxville